Puberty for Tween Girls

"7" Simple Steps to Growing Up Confidently, Celebrating Your Body Changes, and Mastering Puberty

---

The Mentor Bucket

Table of Contents

Introduction

"Today you are You, that is truer than true. There is no one alive who is Youer than You."
Dr. Seuss

Hey, amazing girl!

Have you ever looked in the mirror and noticed many new changes in your body? Perhaps you now have pimples, your favorite clothes are getting tighter and no longer fit, or you look taller than a few weeks ago. Maybe you notice a sudden change in your emotions—one minute, you're laughing uncontrollably with your family, and the next, you want to shut the door and avoid everyone at home.

If any of these sounds familiar, don't worry—these changes are all part of growing up. It can feel like they came out of nowhere, leaving you confused, scared, and wondering what's wrong with you. Well, you're beginning an amazing journey called puberty, and all the changes you're experiencing are a result of it.

During puberty, your body will grow and change in ways you never imagined. Your emotions will feel like a rollercoaster as you start seeing yourself and the world differently.

The good news is that all of this is normal and part of the growing-up phase; soon, you'll understand it better.

Yes, puberty can make you feel overwhelmed at times but know that you aren't alone. Everyone goes through puberty before becoming a full-grown woman; your mom, older sister, friends, and even your female teachers at school have all experienced it.

With so many changes happening all at once, it's absolutely normal to have many questions and feel worried. Perhaps you're worried about why your favorite dress doesn't fit anymore, what you should do about those pesky pimples, or why your mood seems to shift too quickly. These worries can be overwhelming, making you feel isolated, and it might seem like no one truly understands what you're going through. But guess what? I totally get it because I've been there and done that!

Puberty can feel like a big, tangled mess of changes, but I'm here to share in that mess and provide answers to the many questions you have.

When I was your age, I wished I had a big sister to guide me through the changes I was experiencing and provide answers to my questions. I imagined what it would've felt like to have someone who could always share her stories, be there to listen to me without judgment, and offer valuable advice. Honestly, having such a support system would've made a significant difference for me.

Unfortunately, I didn't have that figure in my life, and there were times I often felt misunderstood by my parents. They tried their best to be there and support me, but it seemed like they'd forgotten what it felt like to be a tween. I was young and processed things differently than they did.

So, I felt mostly misunderstood; I had to figure many

things out on my own and learn along the way. No doubt, I made plenty of mistakes as I went along, but through each mistake, I learned and became a better version of myself.

If you're like my old self – who didn't have much support and had so many questions buzzing around in my head that even mom or dad couldn't give the right answers to – see me as your big sister who knows it all when it comes to puberty.

I've been through it all before, and I know how it feels when you can't recognize the person staring back at you in the mirror or when your emotions seem out of control. Well, I am here to be your companion and guide you through each step of the way.

Whether you're nervous, excited, or confused right now, every feeling you have is valid, and every question you ask is important. I'll be here to walk you through, providing the answers you need and the support you deserve.

We'll take it one step at a time, starting with the basics of puberty to help you understand what, when, and how puberty starts, demystifying myths surrounding this transformational phase.

You'll learn about the physical changes that come with puberty – increased height, developed curves, bigger breasts – and understand your menstrual cycle. We'll discuss how to manage these changes and take care of your body with good hygiene practices you should maintain. Understanding these changes and why they happen will help you embrace them with a sense of understanding rather than worry.

You'll also find tips on how to handle the emotional ups and downs you're experiencing, providing you with the right strategies to manage these feelings and reassuring you that it's completely normal to have all of them.

No human should be an island; we all need someone to understand us and share our burdens. And because you're not alone in this, we'll discuss how to connect with your parents, friends, and other trusted adults to support you in this journey.

As you read, you'll discover that every girl experiences puberty differently, and that's fine. You are unique, and your journey mustn't be like that of others. This book will show you better ways to love yourself and feel more prepared for what's ahead.

Puberty is a journey we must all take, and this book will prepare you for what's to come. Ready to start this expedition with me?

This is your journey; it's time to own it!

Step 1

Understanding the Basics of Puberty

"Embrace the glorious mess that you are."
Elizabeth Gilbert

Puberty? How does it relate to what I am experiencing?

This was my response when my parents told me that the changes I was experiencing were a result of puberty.

Like my old self, you might feel confused or awkward when you hear the word "puberty." Perhaps you're already experiencing puberty, so you're curious and nervous about the changes happening to your body. Well, puberty is nothing to be scared of or worried about. It is a transformative time in your life that shows you are growing.

Just as Elizabeth Gilbert's quote suggests, there's beauty and wonder in the process of growing up. Embracing the "glorious mess" means that the awkward changes during puberty are a natural part of your journey toward becoming a grown woman.

I remember when I was twelve, I noticed something surprising. One morning, I woke up and noticed that my favorite jeans were now a bit tighter than usual, and it seemed like I had grown taller overnight. Not only that, but I had small bumps on my chest that I hadn't noticed before. At first, I freaked out because I didn't know what was happening and why. *Could something be wrong with me? Was I the only one experiencing these changes?*

After speaking with my parents about the sudden changes I was noticing, I got to understand that I was beginning my journey of puberty, just as millions of other girls around the world were.

Puberty is a time when our body starts to change and grow. Yes, these changes might seem sudden and unexpected, but they are completely normal; it's just a natural part of growing up. Though it might happen at different times and in different ways for each girl, everyone goes through puberty.

This chapter will help you learn about puberty—why it happens and when and how it starts. And it will demystify some common myths surrounding puberty. Knowing these things will prepare you for the journey ahead, and you can know what to expect.

What Is Puberty?

Puberty is an essential phase of growing up that we all experience to help us transition from childhood to adulthood. For young girls, puberty can occur earlier or later, which is completely normal since we are all different. During this time, your body will experience different changes that are driven by hormones.

These hormones are special chemicals in our bodies that act as messengers, telling our bodies to grow and change in new ways. An example of such a hormone is estrogen. This hormone triggers the development of secondary characteristics and prepares your body for reproduction. Besides these changes, you also get to experience new emotions and start seeing the world differently. Are you now more concerned about what you wear and care about how people see you outside? Well, that's puberty at play.

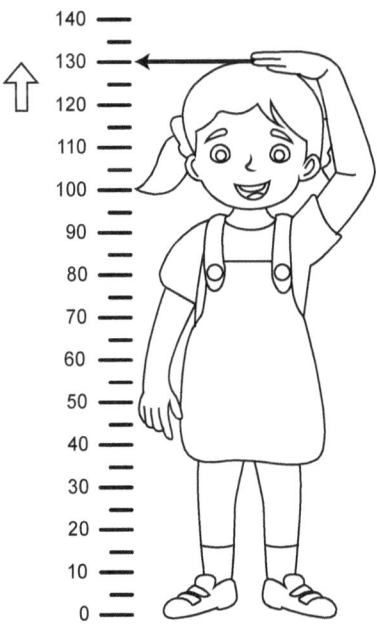

Height Increment

When you understand how puberty works, you will feel more comfortable and confident about handling the changes that come with it. Now, let's discuss when puberty starts.

When Does Puberty Start?

Surprisingly, puberty doesn't have a set year that it starts; it comes at different times for everyone. Typically, it arrives between the ages of 8 and 13 for girls. This variation in the start time is normal, and there's no right time for anyone. We are all unique, have different bodies, and are exposed to several factors that can influence when puberty starts.

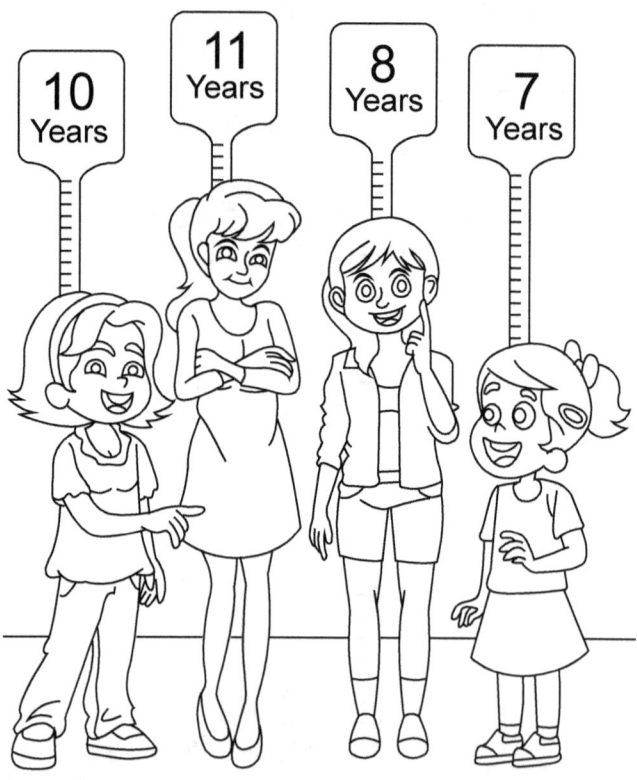

Different Timings of Puberty

Overall, here are some factors influencing when puberty starts:

● **Health and Nutrition**

Your health and nutrition intake play a crucial role in preparing your body for puberty. You'll need to feed your body with a well-balanced diet rich in nutrients to provide your body with the energy it needs. Besides a well-balanced diet, you'll need to maintain a healthy lifestyle that involves regular exercise and adequate sleep. With these, your body will have the right resources to produce the hormones that are crucial for starting puberty.

● **Genetics**

Your genetic makeup can determine when puberty starts for you. Genes inherited from your family can significantly influence the production of hormones that trigger puberty. Ask around to know whether your mom, older sister, and other female relatives started puberty early or late. There's a high chance for you to follow a similar timeline.

● **Environment**

Environmental factors such as exposure to endocrine-disrupting chemicals found in plastics or pesticides can also affect puberty timing. Certain living conditions such as stress levels and socioeconomic status can indirectly influence hormonal balance and puberty timing.

● **Body Fat**

A certain amount of body fat is needed to support hormonal changes influencing puberty. If you're very athletic or have restrictive eating habits, you'll likely have lower levels of body fat, causing a delay in the onset of puberty. Conversely, high levels of body fat allow fatty tissue to produce the hormones that influence reproductive development, and this can lead to early puberty.

That's it for factors influencing puberty. Next, we'll discuss looking out for the signs that signal the start of puberty.

Though puberty can start at different times, there are certain signs to look out for to indicate its start. These include breast development, body odor, menstruation, and body hair growth. Remember, everyone sees the changes at different times, and it's okay to start earlier or later than your friends.

If you're older than twelve and you're curious or worried about when you'll start puberty, it's best to reach out to a trusted adult. This can be your parent or a healthcare provider who can clarify your worries and provide the right help.

How Does Puberty Start

Puberty kickstarts by bringing different changes in your body, guided by hormones. These changes can be physical, emotional, and social; understanding them will help you know what to expect and get you prepared for this overwhelming phase of growing up.

Let's start with discussing the physical changes you'll likely experience as you enter the puberty phase.

Physical Changes

Puberty starts with signals from the brain, particularly the hypothalamus. This part instructs the pituitary glands to release hormones such as estrogen and progesterone. As a result, you get to experience changes such as:

Skin Changes: During puberty, there's an increased hormone activity, causing alterations in your skin. As your oil glands become more active, you'll likely get oilier skin, resulting in acne and pimples. Yes, these changes can be frustrating, but don't worry; you can manage the changes with proper skin care and hygiene.

Growth Spurts: Most girls will notice a sudden surge in height as they start puberty. If you're quickly outgrowing your clothes, that's an indication that your bones are growing—a clear sign of puberty.

Breast Development: A budding breast is the earliest sign of puberty. As you enter puberty, you'll likely have small lumps on your chest known as breasts. From beneath the nipple, they gradually develop into fuller breasts over time.

Body Hair: I believe you've noticed hair growth in new places such as your pubic area and underarms. Well, that's one of the physical changes that come with puberty, so it's nothing to be worried about.

Menstruation: Have you ever heard someone say they've gotten their period? Menstruation, also referred to as "getting your period," is one of the most significant physical changes you'll experience in puberty, as it shows your reproductive capability as a young girl. This usually starts a few years after puberty, and the timing differs for every girl. If you've not started your period yet, let me give you a heads-up—it can be a bit messy and daunting for you. However, in the next chapter, I'll be sharing everything you need to know about menstruation and providing useful tips to help you manage this natural process.

And that's it for the physical changes! So far, the changes we've discussed are all part of your transformational journey from being a young tween to becoming a full-grown woman. Ensure you embrace them.

Emotional Changes

Besides physical changes, you also get to experience different emotional changes as your body adjusts to fluctuating hormone levels during puberty. Some of these changes include:

Mood Swings: Have you ever been happy and smiling one minute, and then you feel like crying for no reason? You start wondering if something is wrong with you. During puberty, you get to experience a rollercoaster of emotions, from highs to sudden lows, and it's normal to feel this way. Though you don't have much control over these sudden mood swings, they're a result of fluctuating hormone levels in puberty. While this experience can be overwhelming, don't be hard on yourself; it's just a temporary phase in this transformational process.

Increased Sensitivity: Have you noticed you're now more sensitive to the world around you? As your body is changing, you'll begin to experience a shift in your perception of things by becoming more attuned to small changes in your environment and how others see you. Though the increased sensitivity will make you feel more vulnerable, it's also an opportunity to grow and be more self-aware.

Developing a Sense of Identity: During puberty, as never before, you'll be more interested in exploring and defining who you are, your values, beliefs, and interests. This is you, going through self-discovery and laying the foundation for who you'll become as an adult. When you notice these changes, ensure you embrace the opportunity to explore your passion and strengths to build a sense of self that resonates with you.

Social Changes

Certain changes experienced during puberty can impact your relationships and interactions with others. They include:

Changing Relationships: Do you see yourself seeking more privacy and independence and starting to set boundaries with people? During this phase, your relationship with family and friends will likely change. This is a result of your growing independence and evolving sense of self, affecting how you relate with those around you. Though the changes might lead to misunderstandings or conflicts, they're a natural part of growing up and becoming self-reliant.

New Interests: Have you been drawn to new hobbies, activities, and interests that spark your curiosity and make you want to explore the world around you? In the puberty phase, you'll pick an interest in new things, such as discovering a passion for art, music, sports, and even literature. These new interests can provide opportunities for self-expression and personal growth, so embrace the opportunity to express them, and don't be afraid to try out new things or step out of your comfort zone.

Peer Influence: Your friends and peers will likely take on a significant role in your life during puberty. More than ever before, you'll start allowing their behaviors, opinions, and attitudes to have a great impact on your actions and choices. Yes, it's natural to want to fit in or seek to be liked by your peers. However, you must stay true to yourself and your values. Ensure you surround yourself with friends who motivate, uplift, and support you rather than those who bring you down at any opportunity. Don't be afraid to do things your way or to stay apart from the crowd.

Remember, you matter most! It's okay to prioritize your happiness and well-being as you navigate puberty. Be open to exploring new interests and experiences; build relationships that nurture and empower you.

Puberty isn't just a time to experience difficult emotions. It's a time for growth and discovery in all aspects of your life. Each step you climb will bring you closer to the wonderful girl you're meant to be!

So, as you start this journey, be aware of the changes you're already experiencing or about to experience. Despite puberty being a normal and natural part of the progression toward adulthood, here are a few points you should always remember:

- **Everyone's timeline is different**
When it comes to puberty, there is no one-size-fits-all timeline. While some girls might start earlier, others begin much later, and that's perfectly okay! Don't stress yourself by worrying over things; your body will grow at its own pace, and there will be other factors that can influence when you start puberty. So, if you haven't started, be patient and embrace your individuality; there's definitely no right or wrong time for puberty to start. However, if you're over 15 and haven't noticed signs of puberty, speak to an adult, and together you can see a doctor to discuss your concerns.

- **Embrace growth**
Puberty is a time for significant growth, both physically, emotionally, and socially. When you understand the process and the changes to expect, you can handle any challenges that come your way during this process. Don't be shy about the changes you're experiencing; they are steps bringing you closer to becoming a beautiful young woman.

- **Share your thoughts**

If you have any concerns or questions about the changes you're experiencing, don't hesitate to talk to a trusted adult for guidance and support. They've been through this phase before and have the experience to share what has worked for them with you. So, be open and honest when sharing your thoughts.

- **Take care of yourself**

As you're experiencing or anticipating different changes in your body, don't push self-care under the rug. It's important that you take care of yourself by maintaining a well-balanced diet, exercising regularly, and practicing good hygiene. Pay attention to your body's needs and what it's telling you so you'll know how to serve your body best and get optimal results.

Demystifying Common Myths Surrounding Puberty

Today, information is just a click away, making it easier to access certain knowledge. However, with countless blogs, articles, YouTube videos, and social media posts, you can easily feel overwhelmed just by the sheer volume of advice and stories about puberty.

Since it's difficult to sieve through all this information and know which is right and which is wrong when it comes to changes happening in your body, let's clear up some common myths to help you understand puberty better and feel more confident as you go through this important phase of your life.

Myth 1: Puberty starts at the same age for everyone.

Truth: As mentioned earlier, there is no one-size-fits-all timeline for puberty; everyone starts at different times. However, girls typically start between the ages of 8 and 13. It's normal to start earlier or later than your friends, so stick to your body's schedule.

Myth 2: You can be in control of when puberty starts.

Truth: The onset of puberty isn't something you can control. In fact, it's largely determined by genetics. While eating healthily and staying active are good for your overall well-being, these won't influence when puberty starts.

Myth 3: Emotional changes are only for girls.

Truth: Both girls and boys experience emotional changes during puberty, and it doesn't mean that you're weak. Increased sensitivity, mood swings, and changes in how you feel about yourself are common experiences for everyone going through puberty.

Myth 4: Having acne is a sign of poor hygiene.

Truth: Acne is a normal part of puberty that many girls experience due to an increased level of oil production in the skin. Good hygiene can help you manage acne, but that still doesn't mean having it is a sign of uncleanliness. Regardless of hygiene habits, many girls experience acne during puberty.

Myth 5: Once puberty starts, it never stops.

Truth: Puberty is just a phase that will last for a few years and come to an end. For most girls, puberty is completed by their late teenage years, while for others, it is earlier. Once your body fully matures, the changes you experience will slow down and eventually stop.

Myth 6: Your body will change overnight.

Truth: While some changes in puberty can seem to happen quickly, it is a gradual process that will mostly occur over several years. As you notice different changes in your body, ensure that you are patient and don't expect overnight transformations.

Myth 7: You shouldn't talk about puberty openly.

Truth: It's normal to talk about puberty and ask questions about what's confusing to you. Every grown woman has experienced puberty, and there's absolutely nothing to hide concerning it. By discussing puberty openly with trusted adults, you get to understand your body better and feel more supported.

Myth 8: Boys don't experience puberty.

Truth: Puberty is a universal experience for all genders. So, boys go through puberty even though the changes they experience may differ. They grow body and facial hair, have voice changes, and experience growth spurts.

Myth 9: Puberty affects only your body.

Truth: Puberty can affect your body, emotions, and social life. It's a time for significant growth; when you get to experience changes in different aspects of your life. Earlier, we discussed how this will manifest.

Myth 10: You should be ashamed of the changes in puberty.

Truth: The changes experienced during puberty are natural and nothing to be ashamed of. Every adult – your mom, older sister, aunt, some of your friends, and your female teachers – has gone through it. Be confident in yourself and embrace the changes as you navigate puberty.

By debunking these myths, you can approach puberty with the right knowledge and a better perspective.

Finally, even though everyone goes through puberty, we go through it a little differently. Maybe some of your friends have gotten curves, and you haven't. Perhaps your best friend's voice has changed, and you still hear yourself sounding like a kid. All these don't matter; there is no right or wrong way to look. Everyone will catch up eventually and the differences will even out. What matters is that you are unique both on the inside and outside.

In the next chapter, we'll discuss the physical changes you'll experience during puberty by focusing on how your body grows and develops, what these changes mean, and how to take care of your evolving body. You'll also get helpful tips to help you feel confident and comfortable in your own skin.

Stay with me as you're about to learn more about your wonderful body!

Step 2
Exploring Your Body

"To love oneself is the beginning of a lifelong romance."
Oscar Wilde

I remember waking up feeling uncomfortable between my legs a few months after I clocked twelve years old. Unluckily for me, I was over at a friend's home, so I felt even more uncomfortable. I tiptoed to the bathroom and screamed when I saw blood coming out of my private part.

Immediately, my friends woke up and crowded the bathroom. They looked worried and scared. All of us were young, so no one knew exactly what to do or say. The host slipped out of there and went to wake her mom. It was only 4:00 am.

Her mom looked pissed when she came to find me in the bathroom. I felt bad for disturbing her sleep. When she saw me, she asked the other girls to leave and forced a smile on her face.

This is normal, she said. *Don't be alarmed; your mom will explain further.* She tried to reassure me and supervised me as I washed up. She got new panties and a soft pad for me. Although she said it was normal, I couldn't help but panic that I was regressing.

As a baby, I wore diapers. Mom said I ditched those quite early because I stopped peeing on myself before age two. So, it was scary for twelve-year-old me to return to needing diapers, even if they looked thinner.

I was terrified that instead of making progress, I was regressing. I wondered if I had a terminal disease. I trembled when I thought about showing my face in front of my friends again. *Would they laugh at me? Would they talk behind my back?*

I remember the soft look in my mom's eyes when she received me that morning. She sat me down and held a mini-lecture on menstruation and hygiene. I was dazed at first, but a repeat of that lecture some months later made me feel confident.

Along with the shock of menstruation came the discovery of many changes to my body. I was growing hair in places that were not my head, and my breasts were growing. When my mom told me they were growing to become like hers, I felt as if I'd been living a lie.

My whole life, I thought my mom always looked like that, with breasts and long hair. So, I was perplexed when she showed me pictures of her when she was young and walked me through the confusing phase of puberty.

Her guidance helped me transform from feeling like an alien

into a confident, growing female teenager. I want to help you gain some of that confidence, too, so I'm taking my time to write about some of the lessons I've learned throughout this journey.

That being said, let's start with discussing the female reproductive system.

The Female Reproductive System

This involves the general system of organs in the female body responsible for birthing children. It includes both external and internal parts that team up to produce eggs, enable fertilization, and support pregnancy.

Outside the body, there's the vulva, which includes the labia majora and minora, the clitoris, and the vaginal opening. Inside, there's the vagina, cervix, uterus, fallopian tubes, and ovaries.

The main job of the female reproductive system entails making eggs, handling periods, and supporting a pregnancy if an egg gets fertilized. The ovaries release eggs and produce hormones such as estrogen and progesterone that keep everything running smoothly.

Each month, the body prepares for a possible pregnancy by building up the uterine lining. If no pregnancy happens, this lining sheds, and you get your period. When an egg gets fertilized, it meets sperm in the fallopian tubes and then implants in the uterus, which provides a cozy spot for the baby to grow.

The uterus also prepares for childbirth by contracting to help push the baby out when it's time. So, basically, it handles everything from making eggs to supporting pregnancy and childbirth while producing important hormones.

The female reproductive system also plays a big role in sexual health and overall well-being. So, it's not just about having babies; it's crucial in many aspects of your health.

Body Changes

The female body goes through a bunch of changes over time. During puberty, you'll notice things such as your breasts developing, starting your period, and growing body hair.

Hormones such as estrogen and progesterone kickstart these changes and signal that your body is ready for reproduction. You might also experience mood swings and changes in your skin and body shape because of these hormones.

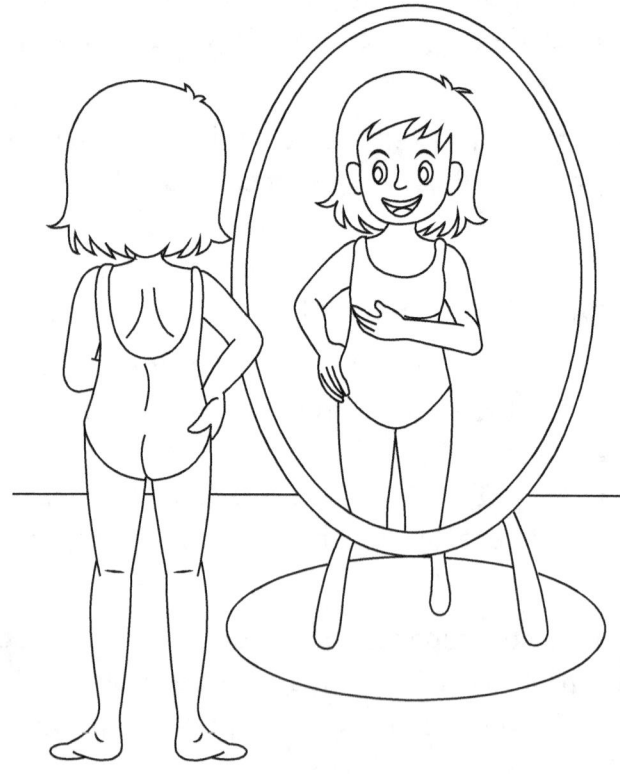

Later on, in your 40s or 50s, you'll go through menopause, which means your periods stop for good. This happens because your hormone levels drop, leading to things such as hot flashes, night sweats, and mood changes.

Your bone density can decrease, and your metabolism might slow down, affecting your weight and energy levels. It's all just part of getting older. Enough of the old age changes. Let's focus on the present.

As mentioned in the previous chapter, when you hit your teenage years, you'll start growing body hair in new places, such as under your arms, on your legs, and in the pubic area. This happens because of hormonal changes during puberty. It's totally normal and just part of growing up. While some girls might feel a bit self-conscious about it, it's a completely natural and healthy part of becoming an adult.

Breast Development

For girls, breast development is one of the first signs of puberty. They start as little bumps under the nipples, called breast buds, and gradually, the breasts get bigger and fuller. This happens because of hormonal changes, mainly from estrogen.

Everyone grows at their own pace, so some girls might develop earlier or later than others, and that's completely normal. This area can become a bit uncomfortable or even sore sometimes, but it's just your body doing its thing.

Just remember, there's no "right" size or shape; everybody is unique! Breast development, also known as thelarche, happens in several stages during puberty. Here are the stages in a nutshell:

- **Stage 1 (Prepubescent):** There's no visible change yet. The breasts are flat, and the nipples are raised only slightly.

- **Stage 2 (Breast Buds):** Small bumps, called breast buds, start to form under the nipples. The area around the nipples (areola) begins to enlarge.

- **Stage 3 (Further Enlargement):** The breasts continue to grow, becoming rounder and fuller. The areola may darken and enlarge further.

- **Stage 4 (Areola and Nipple Growth):** The areola and nipple form a secondary mound on top of the developing breast tissue. This is a distinct stage in which the breast and areola appear as separate.

- **Stage 5 (Mature Breast):** The breasts reach their final adult size and shape. The secondary mound formed by the areola and nipple blends into the rest of the breast.

These stages can vary in timing and pace for each girl, and it's all part of the natural process of growing up.

There are many different types of bras out there, each with their perks that depend on what you need. There are your everyday T-shirt bras, which are smooth and comfortable. Push-up bras give you a little extra lift, and sports bras keep everything in place when you're active. Then there are comfy bralettes without wires, strapless bras for those shoulder-baring outfits, and even convertible bras that let you switch up the straps.

Finding the right fit is all about feeling comfy and supported. Make sure the band isn't too tight, the straps stay put, and the cups cover your boobies without spillage. Remember, it's all about what feels good for you!

Menstruation 101

As mentioned in the previous chapter, menstruation is the monthly shedding of the uterus's lining. It is sometimes called "period," "menses," or "menstrual period." What is shed is usually blood and tissue.

Menstruation isn't rocket science or some terminal disease; it is a natural occurrence only girls experience. Every girl of age sheds blood every month, including your mom, unless she has reached menopause.

The entire process of menstruation was messy and uncomfortable for me, and I always wondered how my mom managed without pausing or being as dreadful as I was. I remember washing myself three times a day when I started, but I soon discovered that menstrual hygiene was more than just washing up. Before we discuss menstrual hygiene, let's quickly see why girls go through this peculiar experience of shedding blood.

As I said, as a woman grows, her body starts to send signals to the brain, telling it that it's ready to carry a baby. It's just like an app that needs upgrading.

When an app is first built, it is in its infancy stage. However, users begin to discover shortcomings, and soon, an update is required. When the app needs several updates to meet all the requirements of the users, the first version is shed for a newer version. This is what puberty looks like, and menstruation is one of the upgrades that girls get.

But why does she need the upgrade? This upgrade is necessary for the reproduction of offspring. As you may have noticed, women are the only ones who get pregnant, which is why we experience menstruation.

The entire process of producing a baby doesn't involve

the woman alone, but it is the woman who has to carry that baby for nine months. The initial body version you had between age zero and age eight cannot carry a baby. Hence, the upgrade. Your body is now ready to carry a baby because your brain has begun the secretion of the female hormones estrogen and progesterone by the ovaries. These hormones trigger the building of the uterus wall, which supports a baby.

When an egg is fertilized, it attaches to the uterus wall. However, when no egg is fertilized, the lining has to break down, which causes bleeding. This is why you should be worried when you don't see the monthly bleeding once you've gotten your period.

The menstruation period happens once a month. But how do you know when it starts and when it ends? The calculation for this period is called the ovulation cycle.

Ovulation is the process where an egg or eggs are released from the ovary. The same chemical messengers and hormones that cause the buildup of the uterus wall also cause the release of eggs from the ovaries.

The egg travels down a tiny passage, called the fallopian tube, all the way down to the uterus. That's where the sperm head fertilizes the egg. If no sperm fertilizes the egg, the wall breaks down and bleeds.

What about the ovulation cycle? The ovulation cycle is the time it takes the ovaries to secrete the hormones estrogen and progesterone, send messages from the ovaries to the brain to build up the wall, and then release the egg.

The process takes 28 days, which is a typical month. When the period starts, some symptoms mark it. I remember feeling really confused in the first years of menstruation because I usually felt weird.

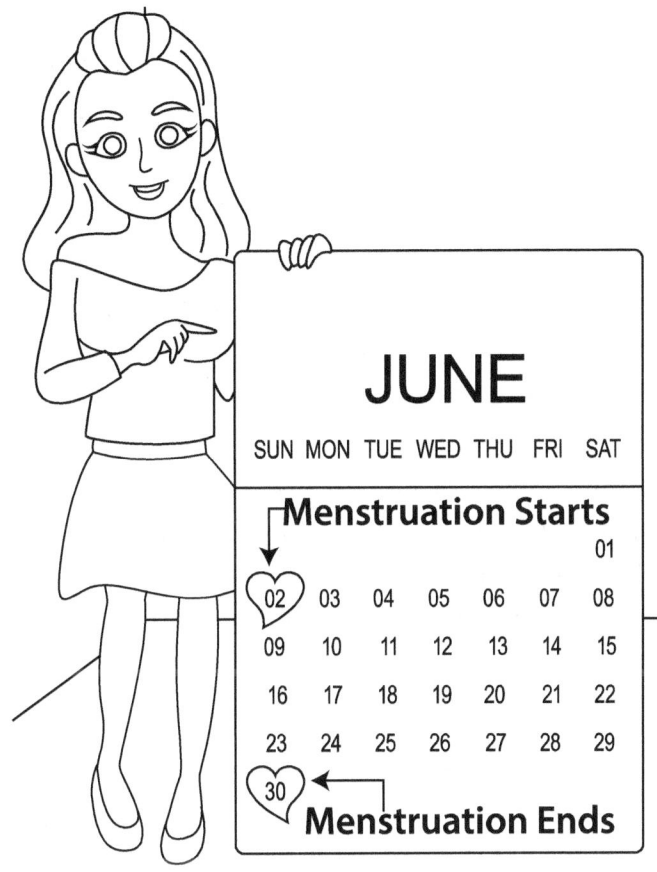

Now that I know better, I'll share some of the signs you should look out for that mark the beginning of your ovulation cycle and the coming of your period. First, you will notice that your vaginal discharge is slippery and sticky. You will also notice that your budding breasts are quite tender and painful. Don't fret; it's just the body doing its work. Next, you will notice slight bloating in your abdomen. Also, you tend to have mood swings and changes in appetite.

Remember me mentioning mood swings as an indicator of puberty? This is likely the root cause. These hormonal movements in your body cause those mood changes, and if you wait it out with the knowledge that something great is happening inside your body, you will handle it better.

To be honest, those mood changes don't ever stop. Even as you grow older and, perhaps, give birth to kids in the future, the hormones still affect your body the same way. The only difference is that you will get better at handling them.

As you age, the effects become normal, and you're better at controlling these emotions, which are byproducts of your hormonal activities. Always remember that you are a miracle, and something wonderful is happening within you.

An average person's period lasts 3 to 7 days, but it can take longer than that. Due to internal medical conditions, some have periods that last for two weeks. If that ever happens, talk to your mom or any trusted adult! A medical practitioner should be contacted for help.

Menstrual Hygiene

The first menstrual experience is always traumatizing, even for people who were prepared. For those who have no prior knowledge of what menstruation is, the first period may feel like an awful experience.

For me, I remember scrubbing my legs like a maniac when I returned from my friend's place. The adults were trying to convince me that it was normal, but none of it felt normal. *Why would I suddenly be bleeding without injury?* It didn't make sense, so I felt disdain for my body. I thought something was wrong with it. Maybe it was cancer or a terminal illness. I just wanted the bleeding to stop, but it didn't. I bled for 5 days and felt immense relief when it stopped.

I thought that was it, but it returned the following month. I remember spending most of the time in the bathroom washing myself because I couldn't stand the thought of a mess and discomfort. However, I couldn't do that forever because I had to go to school and do house chores.

My mom said the world doesn't end just because you're seeing your period. It sounded harsh then, but it's the truth. The world goes on, even if something such as menstrual bleeding is turning your world upside down.

Periods can be painful and messy. But with the right tips, you can handle them better while engaging in your daily activities.

Maintaining Menstrual Hygiene

Menstrual hygiene starts with the food we put in our mouths and ends with the pads we use to absorb the blood.

But what kind of food should you eat and not eat during, before, and after your period? It's easy. When your period starts, remember the three big S's and avoid them. Don't take on **spicy, salty,** and **sweet** things.

Salty foods contain high sodium, and this may lead to water retention, edema, and bloating. This means that fluids get trapped in your system, leading to bloating. When you menstruate, you lose both blood and iron, and too much intake of salty foods can trap those fluids and keep them from leaving the body.

Spicy foods can irritate the stomach, causing diarrhea and nausea. These can adversely affect menstruation and make the entire experience terrible and stressful for you. So, it's best to avoid spicy foods before and during menstruation.

And for the final S, **Sweet foods**. As you may have heard, sweet foods are bad for your health. They are linked to the causes of mood swings during this period. They lead to blood sugar fluctuation, changes in hormonal balance, and mood swings.

Other foods you should avoid during this period include alcohol, caffeine, and red meat. These foods, according to experts, can cause adverse side effects in the menstrual period. They lead to bloating, diarrhea, and dull pain. There's a chance you may have felt some of these symptoms before. Once you take note of it, ensure you watch what you eat.

Now, what about physical hygiene? Apart from eating right, you need to wear the right things, wash the right way, and know the right timing. It's advisable not to wear pads for more than eight hours, but some girls have a much heavier flow, which means they need to change their pads before the eight-hour mark. However, you may not need to worry about that for a long time because, in the initial years of menstruation, the flow is considerably light.

It usually takes two to three years before the menstrual flow gets heavier. However, that isn't a standard period, as this journey differs for everyone. I had a relatively light period for the first five years after that fateful day at my friend's home. So, I wasn't really bothered about that until one afternoon, while I was sitting in the park with my college friends, I felt blood gush out of me. I was alarmed and scared, but I maintained my composure, unlike when I was a kid.

I was a Freshman, so I didn't know yet how to get around campus. Luckily, I had a jacket with me, so I threw it around my waist and began the hunt for a bathroom. When I found one, I was convinced that I was bleeding an awful lot. I was stunned to see the thoroughly stained pad.

I didn't have any extra pad with me that I could change to, so I started the search for the nurse's office. As soon as I got there, a nurse attended to me. She handed me a new pad—new, as in something different from what I was used to wearing. It was thicker and longer. I winced as I took it from her hands. But I got to know that it was a pad for heavier flow.

Several years later, I am still using that kind of sanitary pad, but only sometimes. Sometimes the flow is heavy, and sometimes it's slow. In what you do, ensure you have expert advice. You can always talk to your mom, older sister, or any trusted adult. A little research is good, but first-hand experience is way better.

Best Products for Menstruation

So, what kind of products should you use during your period? And what products should you avoid? Let's get right into it.

First, be conscious that these sanitary pads will come in contact with your skin, so you have to choose something soft and skin-friendly. Go for cotton-based sanitary pads and avoid spandex underwear.

Choose lacey and thin panties, although the thinness of the panties depends on you. If you feel confident with all-through panties, then stick with them, but ensure they are cotton-based or lacey.

There's also the option of a tampon. Tampons are cotton plugs inserted into the vagina. They need to be changed every eight hours, like the sanitary pads. There's also the option of menstrual cups. These are also inserted into the vagina and emptied when they become full. The difference between a menstrual cup and a tampon is that you dispose of tampons after use, while the menstrual cup is emptied when it is full and can be reused.

During this period, there's no need to deviate from what you already do, but you may need to wash more frequently— at least twice daily. You may use skin-friendly bath soap or body wash.

I prefer to use bath soap. I feel reassured when the soap comes off. Bathing with hot water during this period is also therapeutic. You must have heard of the warm bottle massager. If you haven't, it's usually a soft, fancy bottle in various shapes with an opening where warm water is poured. You can use this bottle to relieve menstrual cramps.

If your cramps (that throbbing pain in the lower abdomen during menstruation) feel too painful, you should see a doctor because that isn't normal. You could take analgesics to get rid of the pain or use a warm bottle. Either way, excessive pain could be a symptom of an underlying condition, so make sure you see a doctor.

In the next chapter, we'll discuss the process of embracing your emotional and social changes. It's easy to get frustrated with your constant mood swings, but you're not the problem, I promise. These changes in your body, though scary, are very important. That's why we'll discuss embracing this change.

Step 3
Embracing Emotional and Social Changes

"Change is the only constant in life."
Heraclitus

Just the other day at the annual family bakeout, my niece, who had been bubbling all over the place, suddenly sat still. When her siblings asked what happened, she ignored them.

I sat by the dining table and watched my niece above the rim of my coffee cup, remembering my own moments of emotional change. My sister, who is her mother, reached out to talk to her with a look of concern on her face.

Initially, she was all ears, but in a split second, she lashed out at her mom. It was a thunderous shout, but it was clear she didn't intend it. Her mom, in response, raised her voice, but I intervened, shaking my head to stop her. Stepping back, my sister allowed me to approach my niece. As I crouched beside her, I realized she was no longer a child, and I understood the situation.

My niece's emotional mood swings were the same I experienced as a tween and as many others do. We all have our unique ways of dealing with it, but it's not advisable to hide your feelings away. We all change as humans, and we should make room for changes and accept that they occur in many forms.

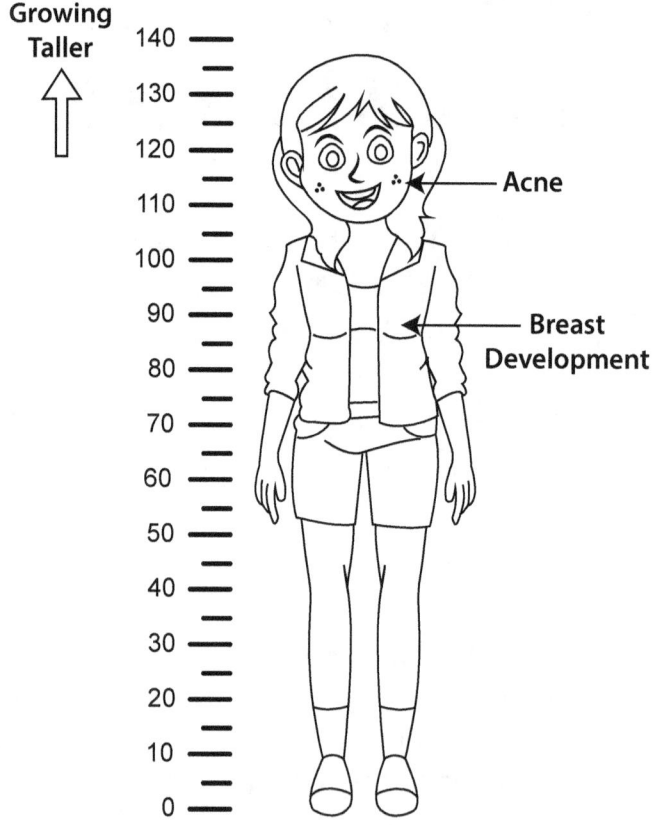

This chapter is focused on understanding your emotions—from how they change to what triggers mood swings and, most importantly, how to cope with them. We'll also discuss developing social skills, understanding and respecting boundaries, and recognizing and tolerating differences in individuality.

Understanding Emotional Changes

Emotional change is the unpredictable act of showing different feelings and emotions at different times. These emotions may include anger, love, joy, confusion, sadness, frustration, irritation, self-consciousness, and anxiety. During puberty, emotional changes are usually highly developed and begin to reflect strongly.

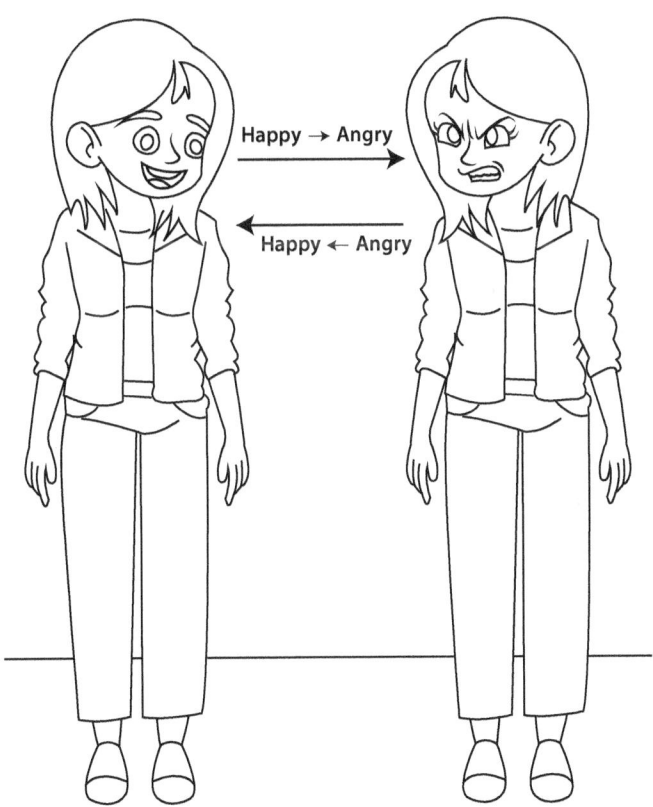

Some emotional changes you may experience during puberty include:

● **Mood swings**
You'll definitely feel happy to do the things you love. For example, when you are playing hockey, basketball, tennis, and video games, or you are drawing, painting, singing, or playing a musical instrument. You can be so overwhelmed with joy that you also feel you need to take a break. And shortly after, you feel a rush of anger or sadness. All of a sudden, you are overwhelmed and don't feel like doing anything anymore. It becomes a rollercoaster of emotions.

● **Frustration**
This happens to the best of us. Frustration is a mixture of exhaustion, anger, and irritation. It can be either short or long-term and is often unexplainable. Most of the time, you feel frustrated when you keep trying something that doesn't work out. As you repeat what you're doing to get the results you want, you can become frustrated, leading you to lash out in anger at others or give up entirely.

● **Self-consciousness**
Do you sometimes find yourself staring for several hours at the mirror, mulling over every different speck of hair or acne on your face? Do you put on your favorite jacket and suddenly hate how it looks on you? That's you being self-conscious. This feeling sometimes creeps up on you, and you become so aware of yourself that you might start comparing yourself to others and disliking the things you used to care for.

● **Anxiety**
Anxiety is a state of unrest that can make you alert and scared. It is mostly followed by sweating, increased

breathing, and heart rate. Anxiety can be a response to incoming danger or threat. While it can help you to get things done when you should, anxiety can leave you feeling unsettled and in fear.

● **Constant loneliness**

Due to the unstable changes in your body and the many emotions you experience, you might find yourself avoiding people and moving back into your own space. You may prefer being alone to being surrounded by peers, friends, or family, and this can cause feelings of doubt, failure, frustration, and anxiety.

Puberty can make you feel as if your emotions are all over the place. One minute, you feel like you're on top of the world, and the next, you want to cry for no reason at all! These emotional ups and downs can be confusing and sometimes overwhelming. And no, you aren't overthinking or imagining things; it's a real change that comes with puberty.

But why exactly does this happen? Why do you feel this way? What's happening in your mind and body, causing these changes? Let's take a closer look at the factors behind these emotions.

● **Hormones**

Hormones are vital chemicals that balance operations in the body and tell the body what to do. Different types of hormones have different functions, but they all contribute to the body's growth. While they bring physical changes to your body, they can also increase emotional reactions and result in mood swings or behavioral changes.

- **Search for identity**

As you grow older, you'll struggle to find out who you truly are. This quest will make you try out different hobbies, lifestyles, or skills before you finally find what aspect of life you're truly great at. This search for identity can make you switch from being full of happiness to sadness to uncertainty to anger, experiencing different emotions.

- **Self-esteem**

Self-esteem entails how we see ourselves in general. It's important because it builds confidence and gives you a sense of self-worth, whether or not you have achieved all you want to. It can also be a form of motivation.

People with little or no self-esteem tend to struggle with mood swings as they have no personal value.

- **Environmental factors**

The environment you are raised in says a lot about your emotions. Kids from broken or dysfunctional families may deal with more emotional struggles than others. Other factors, such as bullying, parental neglect, trauma, and abuse, can also contribute to emotional changes.

Separate Your Emotions

Separating your emotions means understanding them and not judging why you have them. You don't need to avoid them or treat them like a problem. If you know that you get frustrated, anxious, and sad most of the time, before addressing the other emotions, find out why you are feeling the way you do and what is making you upset.

To separate your emotions, you need to recognize and identify each feeling individually rather than letting them all blend into one big, overwhelming sensation.

For example, you could be planning to write a test and also be the best player on the Lacrosse team while also dealing with the death of your dog. This situation can evoke different emotions in anyone.

To separate your emotions, be aware that you're frustrated because you've been practicing over and over again to get that position on the Lacrosse team. Next, you know you are anxious because the test is in a week, and you're sad because you just buried your dog.

Based on the strongest emotion you're feeling after separating, you can address your reactions one after the other. That way, you're not crushed by the heavy weight of the three emotions combined.

Now that you've learned how to separate your emotions, it's time to focus on how to express them:

- **Give yourself time**
First, there's no specific deadline for handling your emotions. You can do it when you feel like it without feeling under pressure. You can seek out fun activities to distract you or take deep breaths when you feel overwhelmed. The good thing about this is that you can always continue whenever you want to.

- **Accept the emotions**
You've identified each emotion now, but have you truly accepted them? Have you accepted that you're angry over something? Accepted that you've been scared for some weeks now? Or are you so confused that all you want to do is scream out loud? When you accept the emotions you feel, you'll become comfortable with the emotions you're feeling at the moment. That way, you don't see being angry as a bad thing or being anxious as something to hide. Rather, you

see them as a representation of what is going through your body, head, and mind.

- **Write them out**

Writing things down helps you keep track. To manage your emotions, you can keep a journal or anything you like to write in. Start by listing how you feel and why you feel that way. You can also find out what triggers those feelings and write them down. Over time, you'll become familiar with your emotions.

- **Talk to someone**

Find someone you trust to share your experiences, feelings, and problems. This can be your mom or any trusted adult. Sharing your feelings with them can help lift your soul and make you feel lighter.

Developing Social Skills

You need basic social skills to interact and communicate with others. These skills help you form relationships, learn, and cooperate with people. These skills can be verbal or nonverbal, e.g., gestures or body language.

Developing social skills will help you interact positively, socialize, and fit into a society/community. Social skills can be improved by:

- Telling stories. You can grasp things easily by looking at descriptive pictures, which makes it easier for you to learn through imagination.

- Playing with toys that involve building, painting, and setting things in place, such as Legos, jigsaws, and clay molds, can help you interact and work with others.

- Nonverbal communication, such as eye language, gestures, body language, or imitation, is also useful.

Making New Friends and Expanding Your Social Circle

The easiest ways to make new friends are by making small talk, bringing up suggestions, asking questions, and engaging in new things together. However, it is advisable to take things slowly and start by introducing yourself or inviting over the person in question.

You can also start some small talk about something you both have in common, such as the weather. Compliment their outfit or any accessory they're putting on. There's no formula to getting things, so it's important to prepare yourself for rejection or lack of interest by some people. However, this should not stop you from trying again.

If you already have a group of friends, you can invite one more person to join your social circle. Before doing this, you should seek out the opinions of other members of your friendship group and ensure that they support you. This is to maintain the orderliness of the group. Ensure you're empathic and kind when dealing with people.

Social differences are the differences between people based on their physical, cultural, social, and religious characteristics. Understanding that people grow up under conditions different from yours can help you relate with others better without causing tension. For example, if someone has a different way of cooking a certain dish than the way you're used to, rather than make a big deal out of it, you can learn something new and also savor the food.

If you're confused about someone's way of interpreting situations, you can start by being patient with them, discussing with them face-to-face, learning from them, and sharing your own views with them, without arguing or claiming to be right. That way, you get to respect them and vice versa.

Navigating Friendships and Relationships

Friendships are conscious and voluntary relationships between people with common interests. It's a bond that is usually long-lasting, given that all parties involved are willing to keep it going.

Do you ever see two or more people hang out daily? Not only are they always around one another, but they do many things together and plan their goals and futures together. That's friendship. As much as this type of relationship is desirable, you need to ensure that your friendships are healthy.

Healthy friendships and relationships involve respect and mutual trust. Other noticeable qualities of a healthy friendship include trust and loyalty, openness and acceptance, growth and support, respect for boundaries, and intentionality and consistency.

Unhealthy friendships, on the other hand, are associated with toxicity, a feeling of overwhelming disrespect, stress, and exhaustion. It's not advisable to hang on to friendships like this, as they can be harmful to you and even cause emotional instability. Unhealthy friendships are characterized by lots of drama, disrespect, control, competition, and bad behaviors rubbing off.

Friendships are a huge part of your life, especially during

the tween years. As you change and grow, so do your friendships. One important skill to keep you grounded and ensure your friendship remains healthy is having good communication skills.

Communication can involve using words, emotions, body language, and so on to send, retrieve, and process information. Communication skills are necessary because they help maintain good, strong relationships, boost confidence, solve problems, and encourage cooperation.

With great communication skills, you can share ideas and pass on information to others. To communicate well, you need to prepare yourself beforehand, write down what you'd like to say in a journal and practice it, not only talk but also listen attentively, try not to interrupt, and, last, maintain good eye contact and body language.

In step 5, we'll discuss how to improve communication with your parents, friends, and other trusted adults.

Dealing with Bullying and Peer Pressure

Bullying is the act of picking up on someone, while a bully is someone who picks on someone else. Bullying can take place anywhere: between siblings, in school, on playgrounds, and even on the internet (usually referred to as cyberbullying).

Dealing with bullies is a process that must involve adults and persons of authority, especially when physical assault is involved. Ensure you report what transpired, and don't keep quiet. Avoid coming in contact with the bully until action is taken. Act confident, but don't confront your bully. Let the adults handle the situation.

Another issue worth mentioning is peer pressure. Peer pressure is the act of influencing someone to do something they wouldn't do on their own. It usually occurs in friendships or large groups.

Peer pressure works quickly because all that has to happen is for the person being influenced to see it as cool. For example, you see a pair of boots; you see that they're cool, and you move on. Five out of your six friends buy the boot and start telling you to get yours. On your own, you wouldn't have bought them, but you did because your friends were buying them. That's peer pressure at work!

To avoid the influence of peer pressure, ensure you're clear about what you want and don't want, set boundaries with your friends, and hold yourself accountable to someone older (a parent or guardian).

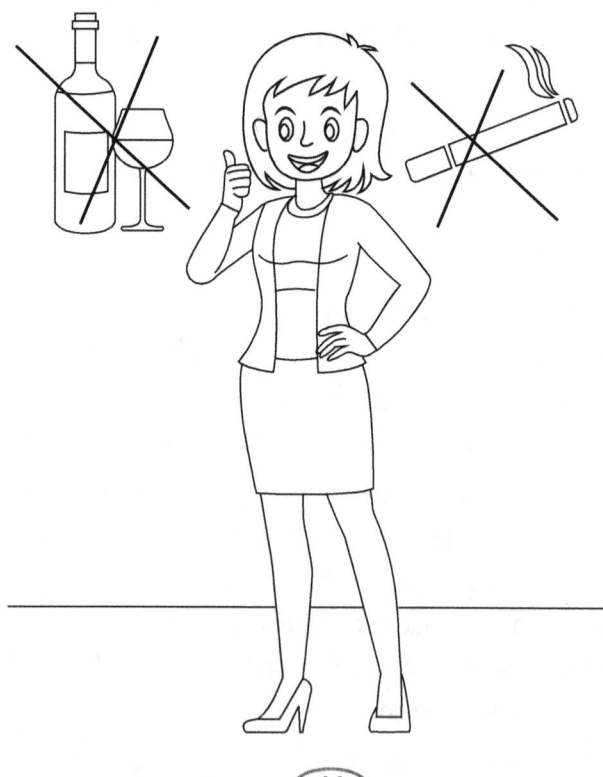

Setting Boundaries and Personal Safety

When you stretch a rubber band, it expands further than its original length. However, when you stretch the rubber band past its elasticity point, it begins to lose its elasticity and finally reaches the breaking point. The rubber band splits apart and becomes unrepairable. It is similar to boundaries, as there is a limit to what you can withstand and endure. When that boundary is passed, it leads to disrespect, and you can even lose yourself in the process.

When people recognize and respect your boundaries, it shows they mean well, respect you, and appreciate being your friend. As mentioned earlier, people in a healthy friendship should have mutual respect for one another.

Understanding and Establishing Personal Boundaries

Boundaries are a form of clarity that allows people to know how to interact with you and what behaviors they should expect from you, too. It keeps you grounded and in control. Setting boundaries is a way of protecting yourself and your emotions. With boundaries in check and unpushed, you don't react angrily or get disappointed easily.

Remember, you aren't too young to set boundaries. The following will guide you on how to set them:

- **Decide on the boundaries you'd like to set**
You can start by listing out the behaviors you like as opposed to the things you don't like and won't enjoy being done to you. After identifying them, learn why you are uncomfortable when these boundaries are pushed and what

triggers a reaction from you. Once you are familiar with these, you can start setting them slowly.

- **Be clear and concise**

Don't set too many boundaries at once. As you set them, let your friends and relatives know so they are not confused. Also, they should not overstep your boundaries due to their ignorance. Learn to say no and stand on your words. Clear communication dispels any form of disrespect. Let it be known what you want or don't want mentally, emotionally, career-wise, physically, in friendships, or during conversations.

- **Voice out when boundaries are pushed**

Communicating your displeasure about a breakage of any of your boundaries makes them clearer to all. Also, consequences should be set to attach more importance to the set boundaries. Also note that while voicing out, you shouldn't lash out by yelling or completely burning bridges with your friends.

Note that you can always revisit, reset, and readjust your set boundaries whenever you like.

How to Recognize and Respond to Unsafe Situations

As a growing teenager, it is important for you to stay safe from dangerous and harmful situations. Whenever you suddenly feel uncomfortable about going somewhere, it is safer to stay behind. Or, if you're already at a location and you feel unsafe, immediately reach out to your parents, guardians, or self-care practices and try to move to a safer place.

Before going out, be prepared for unsafe circumstances

by making sure your phones or mobile devices are fully charged, you have access to an internet connection, and you know your country's emergency codes and other important contact addresses of your parents, guardians, or friends. Ensure you let people know your whereabouts. You can even turn on your GPS location and share it with your family members before going out. Learn a few safety guidelines to use during emergencies.

Ensuring Online Safety

The internet is vast, and even with its many benefits, there are many things to be wary of. You need to be careful of the harmful content that appears on the millions of websites available. More importantly, evil humans are lurking on the internet looking for innocent victims to steal from, prey on, or even bully. Your personal information should be kept secure.

When using the internet, avoid pasting your personal information onto public view. Be protective of your login passwords; keep them safe and secure. Be careful who you chat with or make friends with online. While shopping, verify with a trusted adult before logging in to your payment options.

Don't send pictures or share information about yourself that you don't want everyone to see. Avoid meeting online friends physically because people pretend. You can report any account that seems persistent or insists on meeting up when you don't want to. If you discover any cyberstalking, don't hesitate to inform your parents, guardians, or public authorities.

This chapter discussed changing emotional and social skills, navigating friendships and relationships, ensuring safety both physically and online, setting and respecting boundaries, and, finally, dealing with bullying and peer pressure. The next chapter will focus on cultivating healthy habits. Stay with me!

Step 4
Cultivating Healthy Habits

"Success is the sum of small efforts,
repeated day in and day out."
Robert Collier

I remember the day my school hosted a health and wellness fair. In attendance was a former student who had gone on to become a professional athlete. She was one of the speakers and shared her journey toward becoming an athlete. She mentioned how she discovered the power of cultivating healthy habits during her tween years. She discussed how eating well, staying active, and taking care of herself had all contributed to her current success.

Surprisingly, her story resonated with me deeply. At that moment, I started to point out the many parts I've been neglecting. I realized that taking care of my body wasn't just about looking good on the outside or fitting in; it entailed prioritizing my personal hygiene and developing certain habits that would serve me all through my life.

From that moment, cultivating healthy habits became a cornerstone of my well-being. These habits not only helped me manage the physical and emotional changes I experienced while growing up, but they also laid the foundation for a lifetime of health and happiness.

People practice personal hygiene on different levels; some may be intentional about their hygiene, some don't really care, and others do what they can. It's advisable to put your health first. Aside from ensuring that your body is clean, you should also consider what you eat, drink, and use on your body.

You should also pay attention to how you rest. Pushing your body too far until you're stressed to the point where you break down isn't ideal, especially at your age. Yes, tweens can break down, too. I had a lot of breakdowns when I was young, and, trust me, it's not the best thing.

This chapter will focus on discussing building and maintaining healthy habits during puberty to ensure that you'll lay a foundation for a lifetime of health and happiness. Just as the speaker at my school did, you can also discover the power of nurturing your body by discovering helpful personal hygiene practices, eating a balanced diet, staying active, and encouraging good sleep and relaxation. By embracing these habits, you can handle the changes in puberty better and make a significant difference in your life.

Personal Hygiene Practices

As you experience puberty, maintaining personal hygiene becomes more important than ever. Good personal hygiene entails looking after your body and keeping it clean. Personal hygiene protects you from harmful microorganisms or infections that can weaken your immune system. There are certain practices that you have to cultivate and stick to so you prevent diseases and illnesses.

Here's a guide to personal hygiene practices to help you stay fresh, clean, and confident during this phase of growth:

Skin Care

During puberty, your sweat glands become more active, especially in your underarm and pubic areas. The increased perspiration, if not properly managed, can lead to body odor. Regular showers or baths can remove dirt, sweat, and bacteria from your skin, reducing the risk of body odor.

Bathing or showering helps you feel comfortable in your skin. It gets rid of bad odors and harmful microorganisms that can later cause infections.

Here are some tips to keep in mind for skin care practices:

- Depending on your choice or the weather in your location, you can bathe with either cold or hot water. However, ensure the water isn't too hot to avoid burning your skin.

- Aim to bathe or shower at least once daily. If you engage in sports or any physical activity that makes you sweat, you'll need to shower more.

- Use a gentle soap or body wash to clean your body. Pay attention to areas that are more prone to sweat, such as your feet, underarms, and private parts.

- Make sure the washcloth or bathing sponge you're using isn't too harsh against your skin.

- Don't over-scrub your body to avoid removing important body oils and leaving your skin dry. Also, change your washcloths from time to time.

- Look out for a fragrance-free, lightweight, and non-comedogenic moisturizer for your body.

- Use a sunscreen that contains a physical blocker, such as zinc oxide.

- You can use deodorants and antiperspirants to manage your sweat and body odor. While deodorants mask odor, antiperspirants reduce the amount of sweat produced by your glands. Choose products that suit your skin type and preference.

- When applying deodorant or antiperspirant, ensure your skin is clean and dry, usually best after showering. For effective protection, cover the entire underarm area.

Oral Hygiene

Puberty may cause changes in your mouth, such as the eruption of wisdom teeth or sensitivity. Oral hygiene entails keeping your teeth, gums, and mouth clean and free of germs.

It is important to keep your mouth clean every day to prevent cavities, bad breath, and gum disease. According to the World Health Organization (WHO), you should brush your teeth with fluoride toothpaste twice daily, use floss between your teeth, and brush your tongue.

For effective results:

- Brush your teeth at least twice daily with fluoride toothpaste. Ensure that your toothbrush has soft bristles to protect your gums.

- Replace your toothbrush every three months or sooner, especially when you notice signs of wear.

- Flossing daily removes plaque and food particles from between your teeth. This helps you reach places your toothbrush can't.

- You can use an antimicrobial mouthwash to reduce bacteria and freshen your breath.

Note that your teeth don't have to be sparkling white or properly arranged to be considered hygienic. As long as you brush well, floss, and go to your dentist appointments, you're doing a great job with your oral hygiene.

Facial Care

Due to hormonal changes during puberty, your skin may become oilier and more prone to acne. A consistent skincare routine can manage these changes and keep your skin healthy.

For effective results:

- Wash your face twice daily with a gentle cleanser that matches your skin type. Don't use harsh soaps that can strip your skin of its natural oils.

- A non-comedogenic moisturizer won't clog your pores; use it to keep your skin hydrated. Even if you have oily skin, you still need to maintain its balance.

- If you have acne, check for products containing ingredients like benzoyl peroxide or salicylic acid. They can help prevent and reduce breakouts.

- Don't pick or squeeze pimples, as that can lead to scarring and infection.

Hair and Nail Care

Taking care of your hair is part of good body hygiene practices. Most people tend to ignore their hair, but it should be cleaned properly along with every other part of your body. Your hair and scalp can become oilier during puberty due to increased sebaceous gland activity. This can make your hair appear greasy or lead to scalp issues such as dandruff.

Because your hair can breed insects such as lice that can be harmful to you, remember to:

- Use gentle hair products to wash and care for your hair.

- Brush your hair out before you start washing.

- Wash your hair regularly with a shampoo that suits your hair type. For some girls, washing once every two to three days is okay, but this needs to be adjusted according to how oily your hair gets.

- Use conditioner to ensure your hair is soft and manageable. Focus on your hair ends to avoid weighing down the roots.

- Stop overusing hair products like sprays and gels, which can build up on your scalp and contribute to oiliness.

- Apply hair cream to make your hair shine.

- If you don't wash or style your hair at home, be careful of the tools used on you to prevent the contraction of transmittable diseases.

Keeping your nails clean and trimmed helps prevent the accumulation of dirt and bacteria that can lead to infections.

Here are nail care practices to keep in mind:

- Keep your nails short, clipped, and neat since germs can hide under your fingernails.

- Don't chew on your nails to avoid getting any dirt in your mouth. Besides the dirt, chewing your nails makes them look messy.

- Trim your nails with a blade, nail clippers, or scissors. To prevent ingrown nails, ensure you cut straight across and slightly around the edges.

- Be careful while using tools to prevent cutting yourself or using an already infected tool.

- Use a nail brush or old toothbrush to clean under your nails. Do it gently to avoid damaging the skin under your nails.

Hand Washing

You are constantly touching different items and surfaces. If you check your palms under a microscope, you'll be shocked at the number of microorganisms you'll see. Because you can't differentiate which one is dangerous and which isn't, you need to wash your hands repeatedly; not only when you're about to eat.

To ensure your hands are properly washed:

- Use clean running water. Place your hands under the water and wash with soap.

- Rub your hands together in clockwise and counterclockwise directions to form a lather.

- Rub your palms and the back of your hands alike in the same way as mentioned above.

- Get your fingertips clean by rubbing them circularly against the palms of opposite hands.

- Rinse your hands and repeat the motions, only using just the soap.

- Dry your hands with a clean hand towel and moisturize if desired.

Clothing and Laundry

Wearing clean clothes every day is another aspect of good hygiene practices. Ensure that you:

- Wear clean and fresh clothes daily. Ensure your undergarments and socks are also clean.

- Go for breathable fabrics such as cotton. This allows air circulation and reduces sweat buildup.

- Wash your clothes regularly, paying attention to sportswear or items worn close to your skin.

- Avoid using harsh laundry detergents to wash your clothes; opt for skin-friendly ones.

Menstrual Hygiene

In Chapter 2, you were introduced to Menstruation 101, where we discussed everything you should know about getting your period. Here, I'll share a few menstrual hygiene practices to add to what you already know.

During your period, ensure you:

- Wash your hands regularly. I believe you already know the right way to wash your hands; you can always refer to the hand-washing process discussed earlier.

- Change your menstrual products regularly to prevent

getting a rash or microorganisms due to trapped heat and moisture.

- When changing your menstrual products such as pads, tampons, and period underwear, ensure that you first wash your vulva and buttocks with clean water. Wipe from the front to the back, not the other way.

- Dispose of used menstrual products by wrapping them and throwing them in the trash. Don't flush them down the toilet.

- To prevent irritation, use scent-free products.

- Wear cotton underwear to prevent bacteria from growing.

- Stay hydrated and rest.

Nutrition and Healthy Diet

Nutrition is a core part of ensuring your body is well-developed, strong, and healthy. As you're becoming an adolescent, you need to pay attention to what you eat. A balanced diet is needed for development at this stage of life.

Here are why you need a balanced diet:

- A balanced diet is not only necessary for supporting the body as it grows but it's also useful for supporting brain function.

- Puberty is another stage of growth. Therefore, the body requires increased nutritional needs such as protein, iron, and calcium.

- A healthy, balanced diet protects against many chronic diseases such as cancer, diabetes, and heart disease.

- Healthy nutrition helps to improve the immune system to fight against germs and diseases.

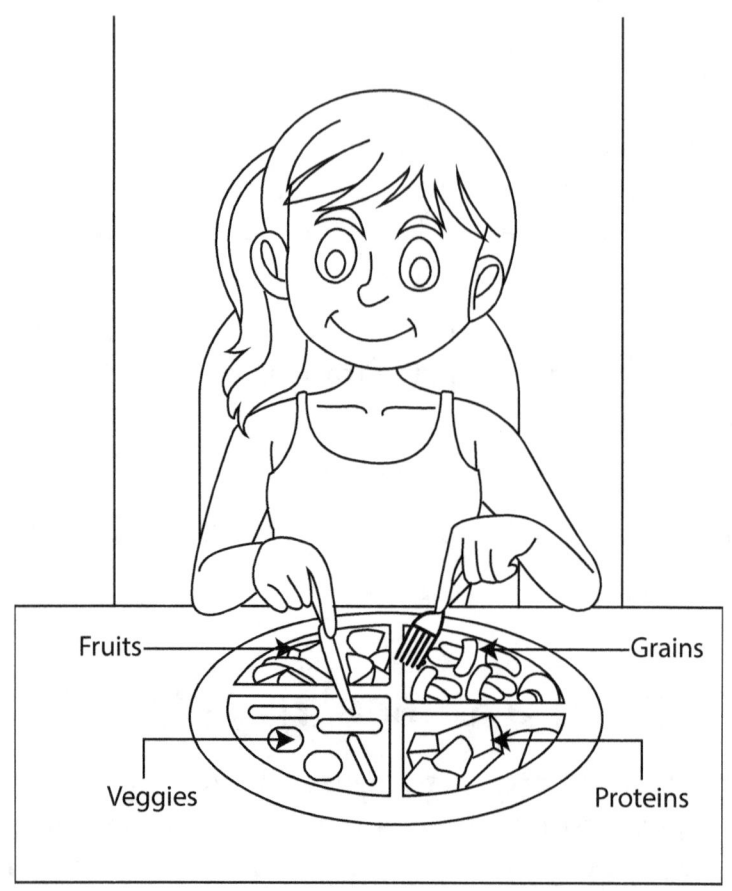

Fruits — Grains

Veggies — Proteins

When the body isn't fed well, the brain can't function well. You need to improve your diet for better brain development. Also, the intake of a lot of sugary food may damage your teeth and cause cavities. This may also result in other dental disorders.

When you don't have a balanced diet, you'll likely have stunted growth and not develop as you should. A low-fiber diet can cause constipation and put you at risk of diseases later in life.

The main cause of obesity is when extra calories are stored in the body as fat. Eating much gives energy, and not using up this energy can cause excess fat in the body.

The higher the intake of salt, the higher the blood pressure. Eating a low-fat diet and plenty of fiber helps lower blood pressure. Carbohydrates have a lot of impact on our blood sugar levels. Also, highly processed foods that are essentially high in calories and low in vitamins, minerals, and fiber break down quite easily and cause a rapid increase in the body's blood sugar level. Not eating enough carbs, therefore, leads to a decrease in the body's blood sugar level.

A balanced diet is essential; it provides you with all the nutrients needed for growth and development.

A balanced diet must include the following:

- **Carbohydrates**

These are the main sources of energy for the body. They contain carbon, hydrogen, and oxygen atoms. The function of carbohydrates in your body is to store energy and serve as an energy source. You need energy to function, and so do your organs. Carbohydrates are classified into three types: fiber (a type of carbohydrate that aids digestion in the body), starch (a good source of energy and the main source of a range of nutrients in your diet), and sugar. Examples of food rich in carbohydrates include rice, cereals, bread, oats, corn, and potatoes.

- **Protein**

Protein is another important part of a healthy diet. It is made of chemical "building blocks" called amino acids. Amino acids are needed to build and repair your muscles, tissues, and bones. They are also used to make hormones and enzymes. Proteins are sometimes used as an energy source because they are to be stored as fat and burned as energy. Examples of proteinous foods are eggs, dairy products, meat, and fish.

- **Vitamins**

Vitamins are nutrients needed in small amounts by the body. But they also work to help you avoid getting sick. Examples of foods containing the vitamins you need are Greek yogurt, beans, meat, fish, carrots, sweet potatoes, spinach, kale, seeds, vegetable oil, and sweet potatoes.

- **Fat and oil**

Fat and oil are essential parts of a balanced diet. Like carbohydrates, fat and oil store energy in the body and provide body heat to keep you warm and alive. Examples of foods with fat and oil are butter, cheese, and lard.

- **Minerals**

These are a vital component of a healthy diet because they fulfill many functions such as providing building materials for your strong bones and maintaining the water balance in your body. Minerals are found in foods such as bread, meat, fish, and milk.

- **Water**

No doubt, this is very significant to nutrition as it aids digestion, but not only digestion. Water also helps to regulate your body's temperature, moistens your body tissues, lubricates the joints, and transports both nutrients and oxygen. Ensure you stay hydrated by drinking enough water, at least 6 to 8 (eight-ounce) cups of water a day.

Exercise

Exercise is an activity that requires physical effort. It is carried out to sustain or improve one's health and fitness.

When we're growing up, the adults around us teach a stereotype that for a lady, doing too much exercise can make you look manly or cause you to become unable to have children. All these are myths and are not true.

Don't prevent yourself from getting fit because you're scared your body will be affected. All genders can and should stay fit. Now that I'm older, I'm still well invested in body fitness. Yes! I hit the gym at least thrice a week.

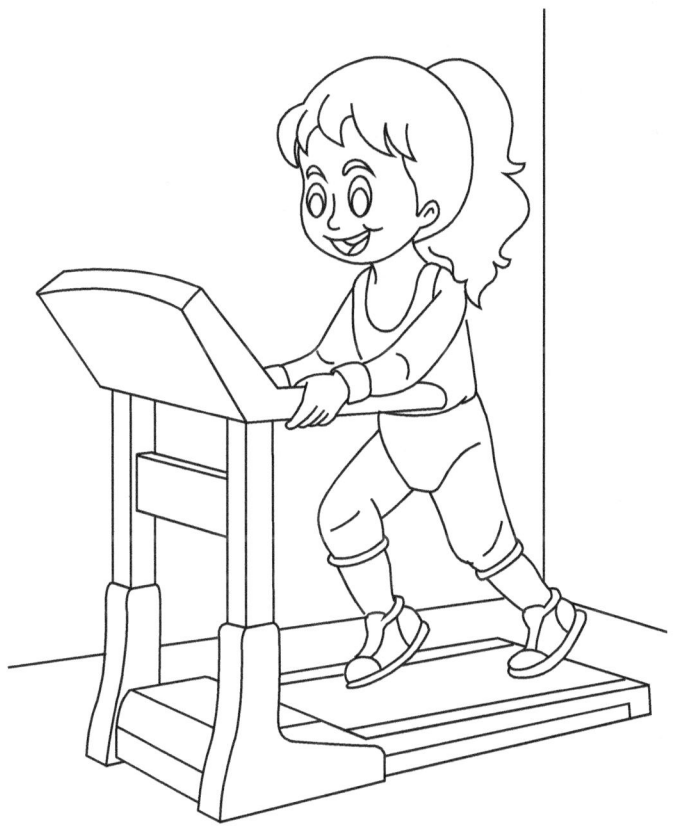

But do you need exercise at such a young age?

Essentially, everyone both old and young needs to exercise their body. Exercise and physical activities can be very fun, and they don't have to be done for long. For example, you can start with 15 or 30 minutes before you increase the time you spend exercising daily.

Here are some benefits of exercising your body:

- **Mood improvement**
When you exercise, the brain releases dopamine, which makes you feel happier. Exercising regularly will make you feel good about yourself and how you look, thereby improving your self-esteem and confidence.

- **Increased energy**
Exercise can improve muscle strength and endurance. It helps send oxygen and nutrients to your body tissues and helps your circulatory system work correctly. When the heart and lungs work well, the whole body works well, giving you enough energy to do your daily activities.

- **Maintaining healthy weight**
Sedentary behavior such as spending hours on screen time, sleeping all day long, and not engaging in any form of physical activity can put the body at risk of shutting down prematurely and gaining excessive weight. Exercise can help prevent excessive weight gain and maintain a healthy weight.

- **Improved health**
Exercise helps prevent and manage certain health conditions, such as high blood sugar, high blood pressure, heart or blood vessel diseases, anxiety, depression, and bone problems. It also uplifts your mood.

Examples of exercises you can engage in are:

- Moderate aerobics, which includes swimming, brisk walking, mowing the lawn, and biking.

- Vigorous aerobics, during which you can run, do swim laps, engage in heavy yard work, or try aerobic dancing.

- Strength training, for which you can run on treadmills, lift weight bars, use resistance bands, and try rock climbing.

Always check with a health professional before starting a new exercise program, especially if you have a health condition.

Sleep and Rest

Have you ever slept and woke up feeling better even though you went to sleep with one banging migraine that had been disturbing you for hours, and you didn't take any medications? Perhaps you woke up, and all the body aches you were feeling a few hours ago suddenly disappeared. If this sounds familiar, it means you've experienced the incredible power of sleep.

Sleep is an essential part of your body's functions, impacting your physical and mental well-being. Contrary to the usual belief that the brain rests while sleeping, the brain works full-time during sleep. The brain keeps everything in check; that's why you wake up hungry even after eating before bedtime.

There are different stages of sleeping, but the best stage is deep sleep. During this stage, your body secretes growth hormones needed for cellular repair and rebuilding. When you get enough deep sleep, you wake up feeling very refreshed.

Sometimes, when you sleep and wake up, you end up still feeling tired and grumpy. That is because you haven't gotten enough sleep, or there's an underlying issue.

How can lack of sleep affect you?

- Lack of sufficient sleep can reduce the rate at which the brain absorbs and retains information. We are always making memories when awake, but sleep will help us keep those memories.

- Sleep deprivation can lead to reduced concentration and make it difficult to pay attention or focus.

- When you are asleep, the immune system secretes a protein called cytokines, which can further promote sleep. Certain cytokines need to be increased when you have an infection or inflammation. This is why you'd always be advised to get more sleep when you are sick. Sleep deprivation may result in a decrease in the production of cytokines.

- Lack of adequate sleep can also affect the menstrual cycle, leading to irregularity and heavy bleeding.

- Sleep deprivation may lead to an increase in negative moods such as anger, frustration, irritability, and sadness. Research has also shown that lack of sleep is one of the symptoms of mood disorders such as anxiety and depression.

How to Get Enough Good Sleep

- Keep the same sleep schedule daily.

- Use an hour before you sleep for quiet time. Don't expose your eyes to light during this period, as this may stimulate the brain to stay awake.

- Avoid heavy meals within a few hours before bedtime. You may have a light snack if you are very hungry.

- Always keep your bedroom well-ventilated, quiet, and dark.

- Limit your afternoon naps, as this may cause you to stay awake throughout the night.

- Avoid anything that has caffeine, such as coffee or caffeinated soda, as these might make you stay awake. You can stick to beverages such as chocolate drinks and tea.

How often should you rest? Eight to ten hours a day is the recommended time for a girl your age to sleep. A high percentage of girls your age don't get enough sleep, and this is crucial for their growth and health. I believe you'll choose to be on the good side.

And that's it for this chapter! I'm sure you've gotten lots of helpful tips on how to look after yourself. You've learned to take your hygiene, nutrition, and sleeping habits more seriously now.

The next chapter will focus on learning to communicate well with your parents and friends. You'll also learn how to open up and build a solid support system for yourself.

Step 5
Improving Communication and Seeking Support

*"No one can whistle a symphony. It takes
a whole orchestra to play it."*
H.E. Luccock

"I don't want to talk to anyone! Leave me alone!"

Yes. That used to be me many years ago. And after saying that, I would shut the door so hard behind me that it would echo through the walls. I'd then lie across my bed and weep for hours, loathing myself and the world alike. My parents would bang endlessly at the door, wait, and eventually give up. Loneliness used to hit me whenever I heard their footsteps walking away.

Have you ever felt alone? Weary and tired of explaining yourself? Or could it be that you don't know how to open up and share how you truly feel? You realize you have also been falling out with people you care about. Suddenly, you're no longer that lovely friend everyone needs. You try not to think about it, but you need to be that supportive friend you've always enjoyed being.

If you can relate to these, then you're not alone, and there's definitely nothing wrong with you for feeling this way.

This chapter will focus on how to process your words and communicate effectively with people around you, from family to friends, as well as how to be a supportive individual to loved ones.

Talking to Parents and Trusted Adults

My parents were not always available, as they were traveling for work or business. It took me a while, with the assistance of my very best friend, to learn how to make the most of the little time we could spend together. She advised me to see my parents as people I was talking to for the first time, but more importantly, to see them as people who will always love me.

Accepting these two principles, the next step I took was to be extra friendly and tell them honestly how I felt. After school that day, I waited for their arrival, and the conversation went like this:

"Mom? Dad? Can we talk?"

Just as my best friend had predicted, they immediately looked concerned and attentive, ready to listen to whatever I had to say. Their expressions showed care and patience, which gave me the encouragement I needed to continue.

Seeing that my parents were willing to listen to me, I took

a deep breath and continued. *"How did you handle things when you were my age?"* I asked, hoping they could relate to my experience. Immediately, my mom's eyes softened with understanding, and she wanted to share her own stories from when she was growing up.

Hearing my mom talk about her experiences made me feel more at ease. I felt relieved knowing I wasn't alone or weird. By the end of the conversation, I felt lighter, as if the weight I'd been carrying was immediately lifted off my shoulder. I realized that talking to my parents wasn't as scary as I had imagined. It was very reassuring, and I am glad I took that bold step.

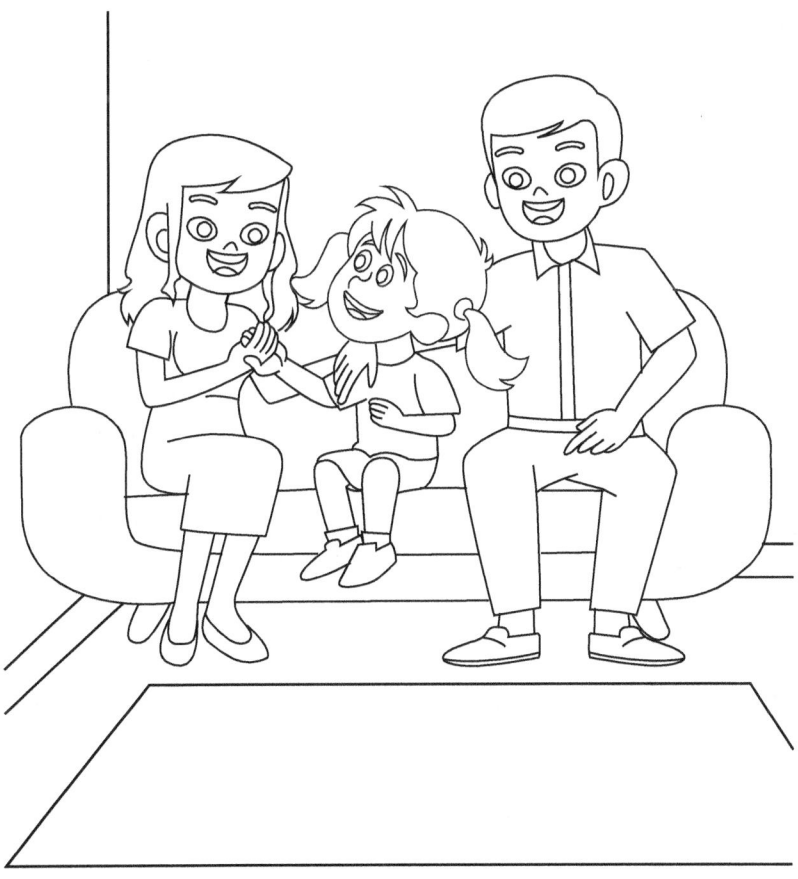

I understand that opening up to your parents during this time can feel daunting, but trust me, it can make a world of difference. Your parents might seem like they don't have the time or understand such an experience, but they've been through puberty themselves and can offer first-hand experience and support. So, if you ever find yourself struggling, or if you have many questions bothering your mind, don't hesitate to reach out to your parents by starting with, "Mom? Dad? Can we talk?" It worked for me, and I am certain it will open up a world of understanding and support for you. Your parents are there to help and support you through this phase, so don't shut them out. I am sure they want to be there for you, just as mine were for me.

Starting a conversation about your feelings might feel challenging, but it doesn't have to be. Here are the steps to help you get started:

Step 1: Find the "Why"

First, the reason you find it difficult to communicate should be obvious to you. Identifying your barriers to communication can help you address them more effectively. You might be a shy and introverted person—angry, overwhelmed, or even finding more comfort in using your mobile phone than speaking with your parents. To discover the reasons behind why you don't communicate, you can get a journal and write down what comes to your mind. Writing down your thoughts and feelings each day can help you become more aware of what's going on inside you.

Ask yourself questions such as, *"What makes me so nervous about talking to my parents?" "Why am I more comfortable texting than talking face-to-face?" "Are there specific topics that I avoid discussing with them? Why?"*

Once you've identified why you find it difficult to communicate, you're in a better position to address these challenges.

Step 2: Listen

Our parents are human and have issues they deal with. However, this is not an excuse for them to fail to be open to sustaining a proper parent-child relationship with you. At times, settle down and hear them out. Ask about their day, what they'd like to tell you, anything at all. You'll be amazed at how much you're going to find out about their lives.

Listening also comes hand-in-hand with the ability to engage in that conversation. Give a little compliment on their outfit, jewelry, or hair, and also include small talks about your day and certain ideas about important issues. Trust me when I say this is the real icebreaker.

Step 3: Don't Just Listen, Look

Actions, they say, speak louder than the voice. Body language shows you more than just words. From a single glance, you'll understand the mood of your parents, easily deducing if they're happy, sad, exhausted, or broody. You can also communicate with them without speaking a word—for example, a thumbs up, a gentle pat on the back, or squeezing their hands for reassurance. From understanding people's reactions, you'll learn how to adjust your voice tone or behavior while speaking.

Step 4: Remain Calm

People argue and express their grievances by word of mouth. Mostly, it is inevitable that you'll get into contentious discussions with your parents. When this happens, you don't have to shout or rain on the whole house with your raised voice. You can assert your point and express your feelings directly without losing your cool. If you are nervous, try to take deep breaths and relax your mind.

Step 5: Address the Main Issues

Opening up can be quite uneasy, and eventually, you might have to face uncomfortable one-on-one conversations. No matter who's at fault or how hard it is to face your parental figure squarely, you need to start by addressing the sensitive issue. Listen to their sides of the story, mention yours, and propose a way to go about overcoming any problems. Of course, your parents will be glad to give you advice and share solutions with you.

Step 6: Know When to Stop

To every beginning, there must surely be an end. There are moments when the safer choice is to take a step backward— pausing so that you or the other parties can gather your thoughts. You don't need to go around the corner or beat around the bush. If you discover the conversation is now heading toward an irreconcilable position, it is better to stop pushing it further.

Now that you are familiar with the process for discussing sensitive topics and starting conversations with your parents or trusted adults, it is great to learn how constant communication with them can build trust and understanding.

Communication entails exchanging information, feelings, beliefs, and ways of life. Note that you can't wake up one morning, see some strangers having breakfast in your dining room, and decide to trust them fully. If that were to happen, it would take some time to fully settle into having them around.

Constantly talking with each other, in addition to spending more time together, will strengthen your relationship with your parents. Do things together such as visiting the beach, checking out their favorite place, or even engaging in an artistic activity. Also, a lot of intentionality is needed to create trust between you and them; it is a conscious effort that all parties involved must contribute to.

Disagreements, miscommunication, and words uttered during outbursts will be hashed out. Apologies will be tendered, and conflicts should be resolved.

Talking to Friends and Peers

It is important to maintain relationships outside your family by sharing your experiences through communication. It is great to be that friend that others can call on anytime to have the most fun or life-changing conversations. To make friends, you need to talk; to sustain friendships, you need to converse and be a supportive friend, and you need to speak when spoken to. You see, it all revolves around communication.

Although it's advisable to reach out to adults concerning some of your experiences, one cannot toss aside the words offered by your friends and peers. Due to how well they can relate to the majority of the bodily and emotional changes you're experiencing, it's advisable to communicate with them as well.

A friend is anyone you would do anything for, and you should treat yours as such. My friend who advised me to converse with my parents is an example of a supportive friend. She saw how lonely I'd become and felt the need to help me overcome it through communication.

To improve how you communicate with your friends:

● Be Patient

Patience means being laid-back, calculative, and calm even in chaos. A patient person knows how to control themselves and stop before hurting others. When you're quiet and slow to react, you learn more about your friends just by studying them. They see you as someone who has the time to be present for them at all times.

● Be Inclusive

A supportive friend is always on the lookout for their friends. They accept all sides of their friends without being judgy or treating them as if they don't matter. When you plan to be a supportive friend, you listen to your friend's ideology and perspectives rather than imposing yours on them. You also accept their identities and assist them in being confident with who they really are.

● Be Respectful

Everyone deserves to be respected, regardless of their age. It doesn't matter if they're young or old; what matters is that they are humans and deserve to be treated with importance. Once people see you as someone respectful, they reciprocate and are ready to hold you in high regard. This also involves learning to give people their space when need be.

● Learn to Forgive

You need to forgive your friends just as you forgive your parents back at home. There are no perfect people, so if you feel offended by your friends' actions, the best thing is to address that. However, have it at the back of your mind that mistakes are unavoidable.

● Stay Loyal

When you're loyal to your friend, you understand how important the bond you share is. You recognize their importance and avoid any form of betrayal, such as embarrassment and cheap gossip. Loyalty also means you can be trusted with secrets.

● Listen

Emphasis is being placed on listening skills because when you don't pay attention, you miss lots of signs and information about your loved ones. Would you want a friend who has no idea about your life because they don't listen?

Besides the qualities of being a supportive friend that were listed above, you also need to be selfless, give good advice, and always show up for your people. Note that while choosing who to have as friends, you expect these qualities will also be reciprocated by them.

Dealing with Conflicts

Disagreements are bound to happen in friendships. It could be hurtful not to be on good terms with people you cherish. But the endgame is the ability to overcome such situations without losing the friendship.

Here are ways to manage conflicts when they happen.

● Find out the cause

To eliminate something rotten, you need to discover the main source of the problem. Ask yourself questions about how the fight happened. *How long has it been looming? What did you do about it? How did it make you feel? Is it a situation you can overlook? Do you think the second party feels the same way you do?*

Your answers to these questions will help you clearly understand and determine whether you really think the friendship needs to be saved.

● **Speak up**

It is not enough to try to find out the reason behind the disagreement or fallout; you need to talk about it. Keeping silent and pushing aside difficult conversations will only ruin the relationship more. It will be a case of digging a deeper hole. To help yourself speak up, I'll advise that you set a date, send a text message, pick a location to meet up, and prepare ahead of time.

There's nothing wrong in reaching out first if you truly want to make things work out with the other party. You can also take your time to process your feelings and reach out at a pace that is comfortable for you.

● **Actively listen**

Recall that no matter how high the level of emotion is, you need your listening skills. Address the issue with an open mind and keep your ears open for feedback. As much as you're aggravated, so is the other party, which means they also have their side of the story.

Start by asking the questions you've listed while finding out the reasons behind the conflict. Then, let the dialogue flow. Likewise, watch out for their tone and reaction. Don't stay quiet; respond using your words and body language.

● **Express your concern**

As you try to settle the issue on the ground, be caring and empathetic. You need to show how concerned you are for your friends. If you discover they are going through difficult times, offer to assist. If you understand that their difficulties are beyond your reach, suggest help for them. Either way, let your friend know you are there because you care.

- **Come to an agreement**

Now that you both know what caused the rift, the best step is to solve it and move past it. The two of you should share the blame without pointing fingers. Don't judge, blame, or toss aside perspectives. Neither should you try to justify your actions—it can come out as selfishness. Exchange apologies and move on. If necessary, the intervention of an unbiased third party can be valuable.

- **Stay positive**

Not all resolutions are successful. Should you discover that the conversation is heading nowhere good and you keep going in circles, take a break. Schedule a time to meet up later and remain positive that your issues can be settled. However, if you still feel cheated or manipulated, choose yourself first. Be aware of when people are willing to sustain the good relationship you share and when they're not.

- **Engage in activities you both like**

Nothing breaks the ice faster than having fun together. If you both reach a compromise, do those things you enjoy together and also go to places that strike up nostalgia. You'll realize that while doing this, you and your friend will slip back to how things used to be without the awkwardness. You can also help each other with chores or run certain errands, strengthening your bond through more conversation and laughter.

Cultivating a Support Network

A support network is basically a group of people who show up for you at all times. This set of people is not necessarily related to you by blood. Your support network can be your friends, classmates, or even strangers coming together.

With a support group, you can help or be helped. A support group helps you achieve set goals, keeps you motivated, and channels positivity into your life and that of others. The main focus of a support network is growth.

So, what's the essence of having "your own people?"

- **For Better Recovery**

Life isn't a bed of roses. There are ups and downs. There are times when you feel so low you can hardly leave your bed; when you go through sad moments that leave you unable to function well. With your loved ones around you, you find yourself a little less sad with each passing day. The push from these supportive individuals prevents you from isolating or drowning in loneliness.

- **For Encouragement**

Many times, we set goals and strive to achieve them. For example, I wanted to be a straight-A student so bad! I was doing well academically, but I wanted the A's. It took the motivation of my family, friends, and teachers for me to achieve that and successfully get into my dream college. If these people hadn't rallied around me to boost my morale, I might not have attained that success.

You'll be surprised at how much a simple sticky note with encouraging words can do for you.

- **For Healthy Living**

People get so engrossed in their daily activities that they

forget to look after themselves. For example, you've probably slept too late for a test or skipped breakfast to rush to school. These times can make you exhausted and wear you out eventually. But your support group can stand in line for you, get you snacks to munch on in school, help you regulate your sleeping hours, or recommend effective products when you start breaking out. Even something as small as grabbing a bottle of water to keep you refreshed is very helpful.

● **Opportunity**
You can get various opportunities to do more from the people who are around you. It doesn't stop at the motivation you get from them. Just by a single referral, you can volunteer at a place to boost your chances of getting into college, learn a skill or two, or access free counseling. This way, you can also help others.

How to Build and Maintain Your Support Group

When you have a strong network, the puberty phase becomes easier to manage. These people are there to listen to you, offer advice, and help you feel less alone. To build and maintain your support network, you need to start by finding the right people and nurturing the relationship.

How can you do this?

● **Set a goal**
State the purpose of your support group and what you'd like to focus on achieving. If you're joining one, ensure the objectives of the support network align with yours.

● **Connect with others**
Reach out to interested individuals, including your friends and others. You can also seek help from your parents or guardians.

- **Get a good location**

For your meetings, you'll need a location that is accessible to all. Also, fix a time that matches the schedules of your support group members.

- **Set rules**

As the group grows, create certain rules that everyone abides by. The rules shouldn't be too tasking or rigid considering your age. This will provide structure and enable shared respect.

- **Be creative**

Add a little bit of fun to the system, such as painting sessions, beach hangouts, and games. It helps to keep everyone balanced and motivated.

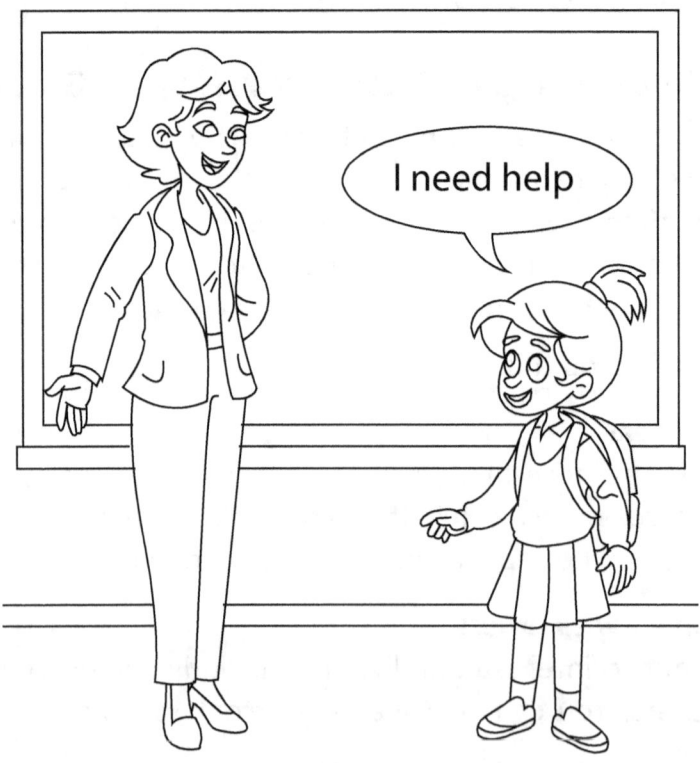

Seeking Help When Needed

If you are in need of help and don't know how to ask for it, or if you need advice but for one reason or another you're unable to find any, the following tips can help you:

- **Reflect on your past experiences**

Why do you need help? Is it your mental health, physical health, emotional struggles, academic frustration, or relationships? Think deeply and write your thoughts down.

- **Accept that you need help**

Most of the time, we humans struggle to acknowledge that we need help, especially when we're independent and think we have everything settled on our own. To accept help, think about it. Also, asking for help doesn't make you a lesser or weaker version of yourself. It doesn't take away your strength from you. Rather, it adds to you. There is strength in being vulnerable because it allows you to let people in so they can be of help.

- **Reach out to your support group**

Now that you have discovered and admitted that you need help, find yourself a support group. Or if you are already in one, open up to them. You can start by contacting a particular member first. Explain to them how you feel and why you think you feel that way. You can also choose to be anonymous for the time being. Remember to take things at your own pace so you don't get too overwhelmed.

- **Embrace the support**

Welcoming the supportiveness of your people is another, different step from asking for help. Asking for help is fine, but you must be willing to embrace the love you are getting. When you do, you realize the value of the group as you start to feel better.

Support can take different forms, and while it might sometimes appear to be too much, embrace it. If professional counseling or therapy is recommended, accept it.

- **Reflect on your recent experience**

Just as you mediated your struggles in the past, you also need to reflect on how far you've gone. You need to compare the progress you're making now to how things were before. This will allow you to embrace more help, adding to your personal growth. You'll see that the support you're getting is worth it.

Now that you've learned how to communicate effectively, resolve conflicts, build or join a support group, and seek assistance, I hope that you follow through with the tips and follow them.

In the next chapter, we'll discuss mental health and its importance to you. You will also learn about stress management and how to develop healthy coping mechanisms. I'm glad you're still reading!

Step 6
Mental Health and Well-Being

"Mental health is not a destination, but a process. It's about how you drive, not where you're going."
Noam Shpancer

Celebrating my tenth birthday was a big deal for me. I wanted all the pink flowers and balloons. I pestered my mom until she gave me everything I wanted. The day after my birthday, I rearranged my room because I was starting to feel like a big girl. I didn't know that being a big girl came with big emotions and responsibilities.

It felt like my brain was running in all directions at once. One morning, I woke up feeling sad. I couldn't stop thinking about all the homework I had to do, but on the other hand, there were still my spelling and math tests.

Somehow, my mom noticed how worried I looked. She patted me on the back and asked me to take a deep breath with her. I took a deep breath and blew out slowly. Shockingly, I felt a bit more relaxed.

My mom asked me how I felt, but I couldn't even explain what was going on in my mind. She then asked me to close my eyes and think of things that made me happy. That was easy! I thought of my favorite ice cream flavor and my best friend.

After some time, my mom told me to open my eyes, and I felt much better. From that day on, I knew just what to do whenever I started feeling worried. I'd take deep breaths and think of things that make me happy. This experience showed me what mental health is. It was then that I truly understood that your mind can control everything that happens to you.

It's shocking what our minds can do! It all starts in your mind whether you're happy, sad, scared, or excited. Your mind helps you know what you're feeling and why. This is one reason mental health is essential.

Your mind helps you think and make decisions every day. It enables you to solve problems and make choices. Taking care of your mind is just as important as taking care of your body so you can be your best self!

Mental health might sound like a huge concept, but it isn't. It's something we all know and talk about—maybe not as often as we talk about ice cream and cake, but if you've ever felt happy or sad, then you have an idea of what mental health is.

This chapter will discuss mental health and its importance. We'll also discuss how to recognize when you feel stressed and share helpful strategies for managing this stress. You'll learn to develop healthy coping habits that support your mental well-being.

Understanding Mental Health

Mental means mind, and health means wellness. When you combine these two words, mental health means a time when your mind is at peace. So, mental health entails ensuring that your brain and mind feel good. It means taking care of your thoughts and feelings.

Mental health involves how you think, feel, and act. It's taking care of your brain just as you take care of your body. Eating healthy food helps your body stay strong, bathing makes your body clean, and doing things that make you happy helps your mind stay calm.

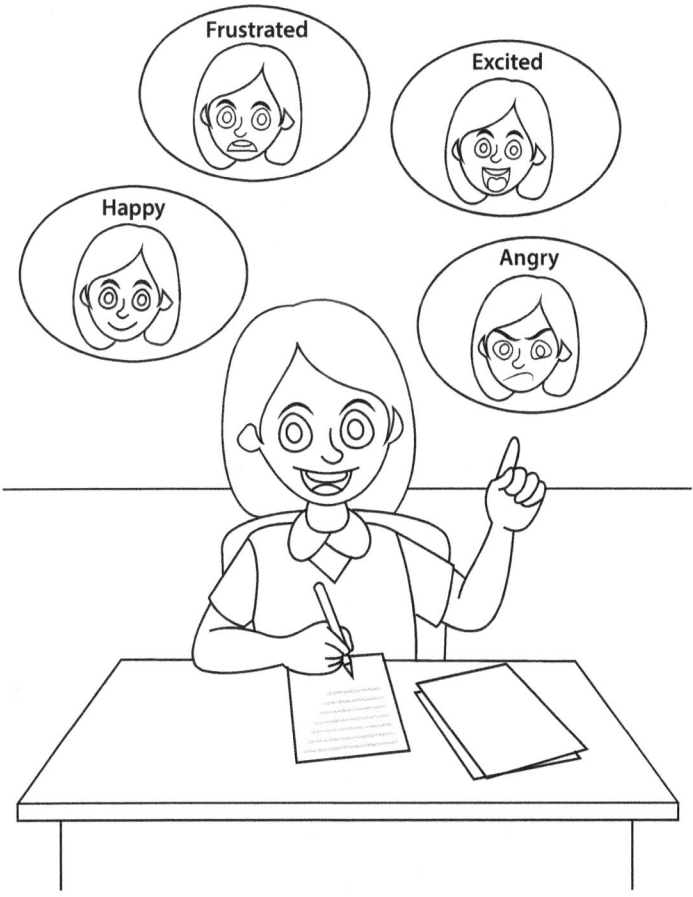

When you're mentally healthy, you have nothing to fear or be worried about. You're cool, calm, and happy. When your mental health is good, you'll feel good and get along well with others.

Mental health is important because our minds control our bodies. When you want your lunch, your mind tells you it's time to eat. Even when you want to sleep, your mind must tell you it's time to rest before falling asleep. Since the mind is so powerful, you must care for it to live a healthy life.

Have you ever noticed that you don't want to do anything when you're sad? Even eating becomes a problem when you're not happy. It's because your mind is not at rest. So, it pushes your body to reject other things. But if you feed your mind with things that make you happy, you'll be eager to eat, work, read, and do different things.

Many things can affect your mental health. They can make you feel sad and cranky. One of them is lack of sleep. You've probably been upset with your mom or dad when they ask you to go to bed early. You shouldn't be upset; they only want the best for you.

Sleep is a time for your brain to rest and recharge for the next day's work. So, when you don't sleep well, you've starved your brain of rest. Your brain will be sad because it needs sleep to work well. Since your brain is tired, you'll also feel tired and maybe cranky.

Getting enough sleep is like charging your phone's battery to the fullest. When your battery is well charged, it functions well and doesn't die off suddenly. That's the same way your body feels when you sleep well. You'll feel stronger and happier. You'll also concentrate well in class.

Another thing that can affect your mental health is the food you eat. I know we all love a cup of ice cream and a slice of cake. However, consuming too much junk and sugary food affects our brains. It can spike your blood sugar, which throws your mind off balance. This is something that healthy foods won't do.

Eating healthy foods gives your brain the energy it needs to think clearly, and it gives your body the strength to carry out activities. Good food nourishes your mind and helps you feel alert all day long.

The people you spend your time with can also affect your mental health. If you spend all day arguing with your siblings, don't expect to feel good at the end of the day. Spending all your time with people who pick arguments and fights with you will only make you feel sad.

When you spend time with family and friends and make each other happy, your mind will be joyful. You'll feel good and have fun. And your mental health will be in a good state.

Common Challenges Associated with Mental Health

So far, we've discussed the importance of mental health; it directs all we do in life. Any problem that affects your mental health affects your entire life. As you experience puberty, you will face some changes that might trigger mental changes in you. I'll discuss what you need to know so you'll be well prepared.

Puberty is a time when your body and mind go through many changes. You might notice that you're growing taller, your body is changing, and you start having new thoughts. Sometimes, these changes can make you happy, excited, or even confused.

Because many things are changing, your body must produce more chemicals to keep up with them. These chemicals can sometimes make you feel happy and then suddenly sad.

For the most part, feeling this way is normal. Everyone goes through it, so you're not alone. All you can do is to find ways to manage your emotions. We'll discuss ways to handle these emotions later in this chapter.

Another challenge that comes with mental health is recognizing and acknowledging that you're struggling with your mental well-being. While puberty comes with mental health struggles, it's not the only possible cause. There are other causes and signs of mental health struggles that shouldn't be mistaken as just puberty hormones.

How can you identify that you're struggling with your mental health?

- **You're always sad and angry**
Everyone gets angry or sad at one point in time. But it would help to become wary when you're moody, unhappy, and irritated for long periods. If you find it difficult to stay happy for too long, and you're angry at the slightest mistake, then you should watch out because you might just be struggling with your mental health.

- **You don't enjoy your favorite activities anymore**
Everyone has things they love to do. It could be singing, cleaning, writing, or any other enjoyment. If you suddenly lose interest in things you used to enjoy, that's a sign that something is wrong. A bigger problem that now overshadows your love for your favorite hobby might be bothering you.

- **You always panic**
Fear is not always a bad thing in itself. Being scared of

upcoming tests can sometimes push you to focus on your books and reading. Fear becomes terrible when it goes on for too long. When you become scared of everything and everyone, you're always on edge. Check yourself because you might be battling with mental health issues.

All these challenges come with mental health problems. But there's still one factor we haven't discussed. This factor is the most important of all the mental health challenges. It's stress! Stress leads to mental health challenges, too, so let's talk about it.

Stress Management

Stress! It sounds like something only adults go through, right? Wrong! Stress is a part of life that no one can avoid. There'll be something to worry about at every corner you come to. Schoolwork, home chores, or personal tasks might stress you out.

I once had a big project due at school. We had to make a presentation about our favorite animal, and I chose dogs. I was initially excited, but as the deadline got closer, I started feeling stressed. I worried about finishing the project on time and making it perfect.

What made it even more stressful was that I also had a lot of homework from other classes. I felt like I didn't have enough time to do everything. My heart started to race, and I couldn't stop thinking about all the work I had to do. I needed to figure out where to start.

To cope with the stress, I decided to take a break and go for a walk outside. The fresh air and the sounds of birds helped clear my mind. I planned to finish my homework and then focus on my dog project. After breaking my tasks into smaller steps, I made them seem more manageable. By the end of the day, I felt much calmer and more in control.

To tackle stress, you first need to identify where it is coming from. What's making you stressed? Is it the many assignments you must submit or the bulk of your home chores? Once you know what's making you stressed, tackling it will be easy.

Before we discuss identifying the cause of your stress, let's consider what stress feels like. Stress is when you feel upset or overwhelmed. It can hurt your tummy, give you a headache, or make you feel tired. I want you to know that everyone feels stressed sometimes, and it's okay to feel this way.

When you start feeling stressed, take a moment to notice how you feel. Are you feeling tense, or is your heart beating fast? Are you feeling sad or worried? Understanding these feelings is the first step.

Next, try to remember what triggered your stress. Did something happen at school? Did you argue with a friend? Was your homework difficult? Sometimes, thinking about what happened during the day can help you determine the cause of your stress.

I'll advise you to keep a journal where you write or draw about your day. You can write about things that made you happy or upset you. Looking back at your journal can help you see if there are patterns. Maybe you feel stressed before a test or when you have too much homework.

Think about what you do every day. Are there activities that make you feel more stressed? Maybe it's a crowded place, a difficult subject at school, or not having enough time to play. Knowing which activities make you feel stressed can help you avoid or prepare for them.

You can also use a simple stress chart to find out the cause of your stress. Draw a big heart and divide it into sections for each part of your day: morning, afternoon, and evening. Use different colors to show how you felt during each part. For example, green is for happiness, yellow is for okay, and red is for stress. This can help you see when you're most stressed and determine what might be causing it.

When you find out what makes you stressed out, you can eliminate it by using coping strategies. Coping strategies are the cure for stress. They'll help you cope well with stress. When you have a coping strategy, you can be sure you have a solution to help you calm down when anxious.

Developing Healthy Coping Mechanisms

Coping mechanisms are like special tricks that help us feel better when we're sad or upset. Think of your favorite toy or a big hug from someone you love. You know how they make you feel safe and happy, right? Well, coping mechanisms are like those hugs for our hearts and minds. They help us feel better when we're struggling.

There was a time I failed a math test and felt down. But then I remembered the drawing pencils my mom gave me for my birthday, which made me feel a little better. I grabbed my markers and paper and started drawing.

I imagined happy times with my pet and my favorite places. Drawing made me feel better because I could express my feelings in a fun way. Each drawing helped me forget my sadness and smile again. Drawing has become my special way of feeling better when I'm lonely or sad. It helps me turn my negative feelings into something beautiful and happy. When I miss my friend or feel down, I know drawing can cheer me up.

Coping mechanisms are those special helpers that keep us feeling okay when things get tough. They help us deal with our feelings in healthy ways. I'll advise you to find activities that make you happy. Talk to someone you trust, take deep breaths, and focus on the good things in your life. These coping mechanisms make a big difference and keep you happy and strong.

You can develop coping mechanisms by practicing the following easy tips.

Talk to Someone: If you're upset or worried, try talking to someone you trust, such as your parents, friends, or teachers. Sharing your feelings can make you feel lighter and happier because it helps you not feel alone.

Write It Down: Sometimes, writing about your day and your feelings in a journal can help you feel better. When you get your thoughts down on paper, it's as if you're letting go of your worries.

Get Moving: Exercise is a great way to feel happier. You can play a sport, dance around, or take a walk. Moving your body helps produce particularly happy hormones, making you feel good inside.

Do Something You Love: Spend time doing activities that make you happy, such as drawing, reading, playing games, or listening to your favorite music. Doing the things you enjoy can take your mind off stress and make you feel joyful.

Take Deep Breaths: When you feel overwhelmed or anxious, take slow, deep breaths in through your nose and out through your mouth. This simple trick can help you calm down and feel more relaxed.

We can't totally avoid stress, but we can cope with it. These coping strategies are here to be your guide during stressful times. They'll lift your mood and help you feel better. So, try all these strategies to find out which works best for you.

There's a strategy that all tweens need to learn. Amid all the activities you must catch up with each day, learn to relax. Just relax! Relaxation is that reset button that, if you push it every night, can help you wake up better and more robust the following day. There are many benefits of relaxation that I'll tell you about in this chapter.

Benefits of Relaxation and Mindfulness Practices

Mindfulness is like a very cold breeze on a hot day. It calms you down and makes you feel happy and relaxed. When you practice mindfulness, you give your brain a reset. Mindfulness helps you feel better when you're upset or nervous, and it helps you focus on your work during the day.

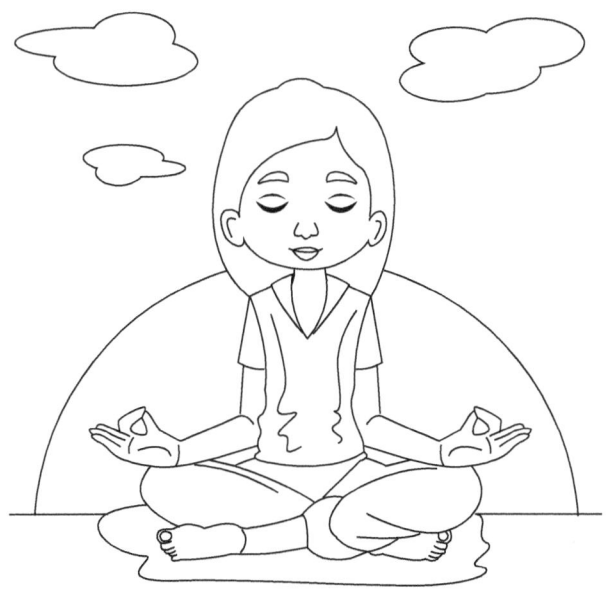

I remember a time when mindfulness really helped me. I was getting ready for a big test at school and feeling really nervous. My heart raced, and I couldn't stop thinking about the questions. But then I remembered what my mom taught me about deep breaths.

I sat down, closed my eyes, and breathed in and out slowly. It made me feel calm and relaxed. When it was time for the test, I focused on each question. I took deep breaths when I felt nervous, which helped me stay calm. Practicing mindfulness made a difference that day. It showed me that staying focused can help me feel confident when I'm worried or nervous.

Whenever I have something important to do, I remember to be mindful, which helps me stay focused on the goal.

Here are mindfulness techniques you can try out:

Deep Breaths

Step 1: Sit comfortably and close your eyes.

Step 2: Breathe in through your nose, and you'll feel your belly rise like a balloon.

Step 3: Breathe out slowly through your mouth until you feel your belly fall like a deflating balloon.

Step 4: Repeat this a few times while focusing on the breath that comes in.

Body Scan

Step 1: Lie down in a comfortable spot.

Step 2: Close your eyes and take a deep breath.

Step 3: Touch your toes and notice how they feel. Are they warm or a little tickly?

Step 4: Slowly move up your body, paying attention to each part—your feet, legs, tummy, arms, and head.

Step 5: Note how each part feels. This is like taking a little tour of your body.

Bubble Blowing

Step 1: Get a special bubble bottle filled with sparkly bubbles!

Step 2: Breathe in, then blow out slowly into your bubble mixture.

Step 3: Watch your bubble float away and imagine it taking your worries with it. See how it floats up to the sky, pops, and disappears!

Step 4: Repeat this a few times till you're calm.

These techniques can make tough times more straightforward to handle. They'll help you stay sane and maintain a good mental state. You'll need to constantly practice these exercises to feel more in control and at peace with yourself. And I assure you that you'll feel better after practicing these techniques.

Now that you know your mind is where the big deal happens, I want you to guard it. Protect your mind with all you've got. Stay away from anything and anyone that makes you sad. Filter the books you read, the songs you listen to, and the friends you keep—they all speak to your mind.

Even after protecting your mind from all kinds of bad things, it's possible that you still feel sad or worried once in a while. That's normal! It's okay to feel all kinds of emotions. Everyone goes through that phase. The best thing you can do to help yourself is to talk to someone you trust, such as your parents or teachers, who can help you feel better when you're upset. Writing in a journal or doing things you love, such as drawing or playing, can also make a big difference.

We learned that mindfulness exercises such as taking deep breaths and focusing on the present moment can help calm your mind and make you feel more peaceful. And don't forget about the benefits of relaxing! Taking time to relax each day, whether by taking deep breaths, doing activities you enjoy, or simply resting, helps your body and mind stay healthy and happy.

Keep practicing these skills and remember to be kind to yourself. You're doing great, and I'm proud of you for learning how to take care of your mental health and well-being!

Step 7
Celebrating Your Changes, Loving Yourself, and Mastering Puberty

"Don't be afraid of change. It's leading you to a new beginning."
Joyce Meyer

When I was young and inexperienced, I loathed some stages of puberty. I would shrink back in shame and fake smiles for days. I even held myself back from pursuing my passion for being a cheerleader because I wasn't confident.

From the way I sound now, you can already tell that I regret acting that way. Although there was nothing wrong with me, I hid from the light and bit my fingers in the dark.

Whether you're short, tall, plus-sized, or slim, I want you to know that you're beautiful and perfect. This isn't an attempt at motivating you. It's actually the truth. In hindsight, I see that I was undergoing a major transformation that took me from zero to a hundred, and I can't even lie—it's happening to you.

All you need during this period is patience and love for the process. Because what comes out of the oven at the end of the day is a body of art, perfect and unique. And when that process becomes a part of you, and you start to see the results, you ought to celebrate.

It's worth throwing fireworks, riding ponies at the amusement park, and hosting a large family dinner. It's a wholesome experience you won't get again, and you will miss it. Yes, I do miss it sometimes. I wish to go back in time and go through it again because I'd know better this time.

My wish will never come true because I can't turn back the hands of time, but you can make your reality better than mine.

In this chapter, we'll focus on embracing body changes. It takes psychological and physical effort to embrace change, and the same is true for puberty. You will learn what body positivity is and why you should embrace it. You will also learn about self-love, self-acceptance, and resilience and how to build it during setbacks. Finally, you will learn how to grow up confidently.

After all is said and done, if your body and mind are not in sync with what's happening around you, then the results might not be impressive in your eyes. But if you train your eyes to appreciate what you see daily, then the results will be impressive!

Embrace Body Positivity

Your body is a journey. That sounds poetic, but it's the truth. You were once a squishy baby, and you grew into an energetic toddler, then an adorable tween. You may not have noticed it, but the adults around you must be taking second glances at you.

Why? Because they can see changes, and they're marvelous. All through life, you will encounter changes in your body; that is why I called it a journey. Think about one time when you embarked on a road trip with your family. You must have been excited at the start, but then you grew impatient, fascinated, relieved, and tired. Those are some emotions associated with traveling, and they are the same with your body.

Changes can make you anxious, but there's no need to get negative about it. Keeping an open mind to all the changes your body is going through during puberty is the practice of body positivity.

You become positive about the growth and disappearance of some features you were used to. You accept these changes as they come and even get excited about them. Even if you've started hating the way you look, you can still change your mindset.

How to Embrace Body Positivity

Embracing body positivity is a journey that involves changing the way you think about yourself and your body. There are some steps to follow to cultivate a positive body image. Let's explore them!

- **Accept yourself**

To change your mindset about your body, you need to first come to terms with the fact that all bodies are unique in their own way. No two bodies are the same. All bodies are worthy of love and respect, regardless of shape, size, color, and ability. Accept the fact that our bodies are unique. Recognize and celebrate the beauty in diversity. Appreciate the variety of body types, shapes, and sizes around you.

- **Get rid of negative thoughts**

Knowing that we are all unique with different body types doesn't make everything all good at once; you need to purge negative thoughts. Though it's going to take some time, it is possible and practicable. For instance, every time you think, *"I hate my thighs,"* scratch that and say, *"My thighs are strong, and they help me move."*

You won't instantly have positive thoughts. You need to practice constantly before you become an expert. However, if you surround yourself with positivity, you can make a huge difference in a short time.

- **Surround yourself with positive influences**

We're in the digital age and exposed to so many influences online and offline. Instead of following influencers who make you feel weird about your body and promote unrealistic beauty standards, watch content from influencers who preach body positivity.

Offline, surround yourself with people and friends who are also actively practicing body positivity so there won't be loopholes for negativity to slip back into. Surround yourself with friends and family who support and uplift you.

- **Practice self-care**

As already mentioned, you need to practice positive self-care. Engage in activities that make you feel good about yourself and your body. This could be anything from taking a relaxing bath to going for a walk in nature, practicing yoga, or meditating.

● **Wear comfortable outfits**

When it comes to outer habits that can help you embrace body positivity, your clothes are a major factor. You need to wear clothes that make you feel good. If a particular outfit makes you feel super cool, don't think twice about wearing it.

It's quite tacky to wear what is popular just because your friends are wearing it. If you don't feel good about it, ditch it. Choose clothes that make you feel comfortable and confident. Don't try to fit into clothes that make you feel uncomfortable.

● **Embrace a healthy lifestyle**

Shift your focus from trying to achieve a certain size to leading a healthy lifestyle. This includes eating nutritious foods, staying active in ways you enjoy, getting enough sleep, and managing stress.

● **Set realistic goals**

Earlier, I mentioned prioritizing your health. That is a realistic goal. Whatever body goals you set for yourself, make sure they are realistic. If you still find yourself looking for a thinner waist or bigger boobs, then you need to watch who you're listening to.

Remember my advice to unfollow unhealthy influencers. This helps clear your mind and set realistic goals. Set achievable goals that are not based on changing your appearance. For example, aim to run a certain distance, master a new yoga pose, or learn a new dance step.

- **Practice self-compassion**

Treat yourself with the same kindness and understanding that you would offer a friend. Forgive yourself for not meeting societal standards and focus on your standards of beauty and health.

In the end, you're just human like everyone else. Making progress isn't always straightforward. You'll fall back sometimes, most times even, but make sure you get up. Forgive yourself every time you slip up.

- **Practice positive self-talk**

Affirmations may sound superstitious, but they really work. Make a habit of speaking kindly to yourself. Regularly remind yourself of your worth and the beauty of your unique body.

- **Show gratitude**

Say thank you to those around you and to yourself. Regularly remind yourself of the things you are grateful for about your body. These could be its ability to wake up, move, create, or feel.

- **Seek help when needed**

Consider talking to a therapist or joining a support group if you're struggling with body image issues. Professional support can provide tools and strategies to help you develop a more positive body image.

As you take care of yourself, take care of others too. Educate your friends and family. Advocate for body positivity in your community. Educate others about the harmful effects of body shaming and the importance of embracing all body types.

All through this period, always remember that everyone's bodies are unique. So, you must celebrate your body's differences. Appreciate what your body can do rather than just how it looks. Celebrate your body's strength, flexibility, endurance, and resilience.

Finally, always remember that it takes time. I'm older now, but I'm still experiencing changes in my body. Remember that embracing body positivity is a process. Be patient with yourself as you work toward a more positive and accepting relationship with your body.

With the strategies discussed so far, you can start to embrace body positivity and develop a healthier, more compassionate relationship with your body. You are unique, delicate, and important.

Self-Love and Acceptance

Mental work is no joke. Reworking your mind to embrace what you see in the mirror is quite tasking, and it takes time, but it is indeed achievable. Here, we'll focus on discussing what self-love is and how to achieve it.

Self-love is the practice of caring for one's well-being and happiness. It involves putting oneself first over others. Self-love is very different from selfishness.

Selfishness involves taking from others, using others, and even abusing others to get what you want without consideration for their well-being. Self-love is taking care of your needs and wants without taking advantage of others in the process.

On the other hand, self-acceptance means coming to terms with all that you are and look like. It is embracing your body – your culture, your gender, and everything that has to do with you – as good.

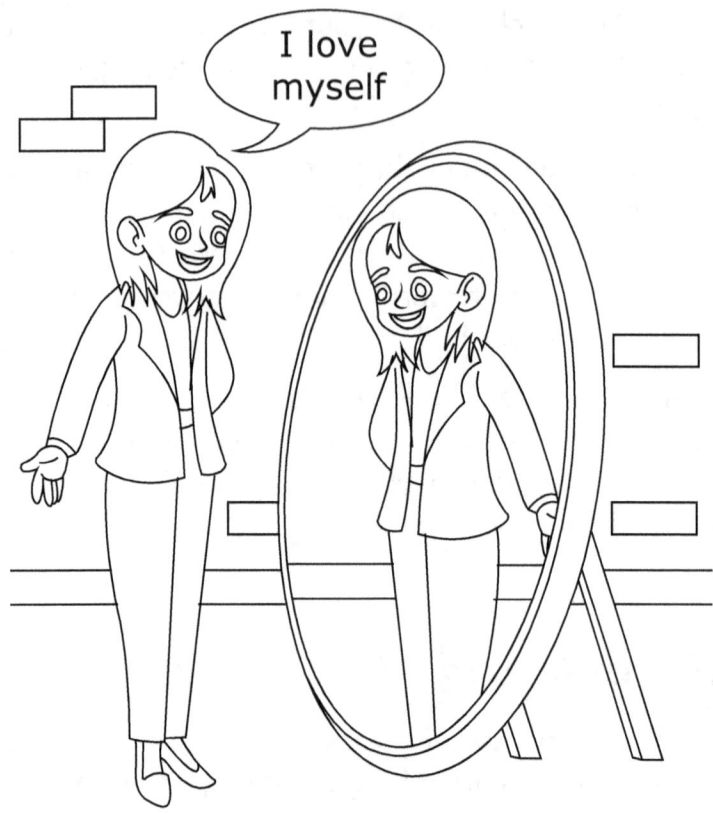

Self-love and self-acceptance go hand in hand. You need self-acceptance to get to self-love, and you need self-love to continue self-acceptance. They are crucial aspects of mental and emotional well-being.

They involve recognizing your worth, treating yourself with kindness, and embracing your true self. I always remind you that these things take time because your heart may be beating fast, and you are looking for a fast resolution, but no, darling, it's a long ride ahead.

How to Practice Self-Love

Self-love involves prioritizing your needs, treating yourself with compassion, and valuing yourself as a person. It involves becoming your very own fan, and here are ways you can start practicing self-love:

- **Make time for yourself**

Naturally, people who love themselves carve out time to care for themselves. Practice self-care by nurturing your physical, emotional, and mental health through activities that bring you joy and relaxation.

- **Be kind to yourself**

And when you care for yourself, you should be gentle and kind. This is the process of self-compassion. It involves being gentle with yourself – especially during times of failure or difficulty – and avoiding destructive self-criticism.

- **It's okay to have boundaries**

Earlier, I recommended surrounding yourself with friends and family who have the same positive goals as you. Now I'm telling you it's okay to have boundaries with friends and family who don't align with your goals and mental well-being.

- **Protect your energy and mental well-being at all costs**

To be your top fan, you must encourage yourself. Practice positive self-talk and acknowledge your achievements. Also, recognize and remember that you're only human, so you have to forgive yourself for times when you fail.

Practicing Self-Acceptance

Self-love, as I've already said, goes hand in hand with self-acceptance. There are certain things you should practice for self-acceptance, and I've listed them below. Remember, it involves embracing everything about you.

- **Know that you're only human**

Self-acceptance isn't denial and isn't delusion. It also isn't abuse and oppression. It involves acknowledging your faults and working on them. With self-acceptance, you know you're human and naturally flawed. But you don't use that as a weapon to be rude and toxic. Every human is flawed, but we all have to strive to be better. So, with self-acceptance, you acknowledge your faults, but you don't judge—you work to improve.

- **Ditch unrealistic expectations**

Once you leave the unrealistic expectations of online beauty influencers, you should begin to embrace your true self. You embrace the dip in your hips, the slight bend of your smile, and the sleepiness of your eyes. They are all unique and beautiful.

- **Be kind to your feelings as you acknowledge them**

To accept oneself is to be present with your thoughts and feelings without trying to change them, but rather accepting them as part of your experience. You are also accommodating to your emotions, behaviors, and thoughts and how they influence your life, without self-rejection.

- **You are just a tween and still growing**

Finally, as I am doing right now, you have to recognize that you are still growing. You will always be growing and evolving. You should also accept that change is a natural part of life. Stay thankful for who you are and what you have rather than focusing on what you lack.

Building Resilience During Setbacks

What I've said about getting prepared for tough times is important, and I'll stress it more here. Building resilience during setbacks is essential for navigating life's challenges and bouncing back stronger.

The following tips on how to build resilience during setbacks would be of great help!

- **Be positive regardless**
I can't stress this enough, but you need to maintain a positive attitude in any situation that you find yourself in. Look for the silver lining and be hopeful. Also, express gratitude every day by acknowledging what you are thankful for, even in tough times.

- **Connect with people**
Connect with like-minded people. Reach out to family, friends, or support groups dealing with similar issues. Sharing your feelings and experiences can provide comfort and different perspectives, thereby expanding your knowledge.

- **Embrace change**
I know that you've seen this repeatedly, but you need to embrace change. Start cultivating flexibility and adaptability. Accept that change is a natural part of life. Being open to new experiences and adapting to new circumstances can make you more resilient.

- **Seek solutions; don't focus on problems**
In the previous section, I talked about focusing on the solutions and not the problems. You also need to do this to build resilience. Develop reliable problem-solving skills and

take action instead of merely looking at the setback.

● Prioritize your well-being

Prioritize your physical, emotional, and mental well-being through regular exercise, a balanced diet, and sufficient sleep. Practice mindfulness, meditation, or deep breathing exercises to manage stress and stay grounded.

● Set goals

Practice SMART goal-making—that is, set goals that are Specific, Measurable, Achievable, Realistic, and Timely. Break down large goals into smaller, achievable steps. Celebrate small victories to build momentum. Keep your long-term goals in mind to stay motivated and focused on the bigger picture. For instance, let's say your goal is to pass math after having failed it. First, don't overwhelm yourself by trying to learn everything at once. You can start with a topic and practice it for a week before moving to the next topic. You can even involve a close friend to hold you accountable and track your progress. Over the next few weeks, you'll see how greatly improved you are.

Developing this skill will not only help you become the girl who handles problems graciously but will also aid you in your chosen career.

● Keep your emotions in check

Darling, you need to learn to recognize and manage your emotions effectively. You are the boss, not your anger or frustration. You're the one who calls the shots. So, stay at the top.

Learn to take charge of your emotions, staying calm and composed in difficult situations. This is quite important because it means not taking responsibility for other people's emotions. You are not responsible for that.

Adopt techniques such as journaling, talking it out, or engaging in creative activities, as these can help you. You should practice staying calm under pressure by deep breathing, meditation, or counting to ten.

● Be confident
Have confidence in your ability to handle challenges. Always remind yourself of past successes and your capacity to overcome difficulties. Continuously work on developing skills that enhance your ability to manage future setbacks.

● Let go of things beyond your control
If situations are beyond your control, it is better to acknowledge the reality of the situation without dwelling on what can't be changed. Learn to let go of things outside your control and focus on what you can influence.

● Reflect
From time to time, reflect on past setbacks and how you overcame them. Identify what worked and what didn't and improve on them. Life is all about looking to the future. You need to think about tomorrow, but never forget to live in the now. Believe that you can influence your future positively and cultivate a sense of hope and optimism about the future, even when facing adversity. View setbacks as opportunities for growth and learning. Understand that failure is a part of the learning process.

There's nothing wrong with seeking professional help. If you're dissatisfied with your progress, consider talking to a therapist or counselor who can offer guidance and support.

Building resilience is a continuous process that involves developing positive habits, fostering a supportive network, and maintaining a hopeful and adaptable mindset. By implementing these strategies, you can better handle setbacks.

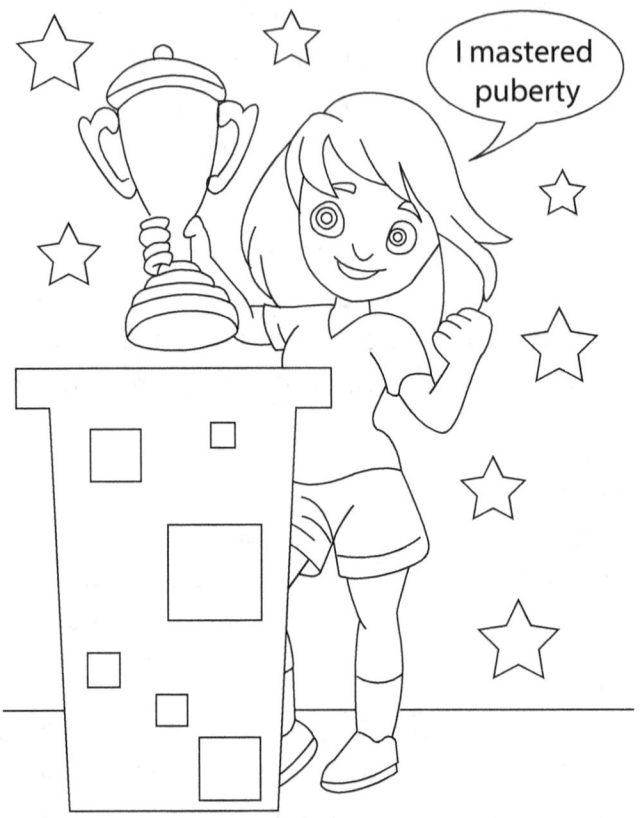

Growing Up Confidently

Growing up confidently involves building self-esteem, developing a positive mindset, and acquiring skills that help you navigate life's challenges. To boost your confidence:

- **Be self-aware**

Take time to understand your strengths, weaknesses, values, and passions. Self-awareness is the foundation of confidence and the fruit of self-love. Tools such as the Myers-Briggs Type Indicator (MBTI) or the Enneagram can provide insight into your personality traits.

Be true to yourself. Embrace your uniqueness, and don't feel pressured to conform to the expectations of others. Live according to your values and principles, as this strengthens your sense of self.

● Set realistic and achievable goals

Remember the smart goals I mentioned earlier? Now is the time to use them again. Make your goals Specific, Measurable, Achievable, Relevant, and Timely. Create a vision board with images and words that represent your goals and aspirations. As you set your goals, keep a gratitude journal to remind yourself of the positive aspects of your life.

● Embrace continuous learning

Focus on your education and continuous learning. Knowledge and skills build confidence. Learn essential life skills such as cooking, managing finances, time management, and effective communication.

● Work on your mind and body

Use positive affirmations to boost your self-esteem. Replace negative thoughts with encouraging ones. Practice mindfulness to stay aware of your thoughts and feelings and manage them positively.

Practice facing your fears, such as public speaking or job interviews, to build confidence. Facing your fears can pull you out of your comfort zone a bit and prepare you for the unknown. It's good to be more prepared for unexpected situations.

Regular physical activity boosts your mood and energy levels. Eat a balanced diet to fuel your body and mind. Ensure you get enough restful sleep to maintain your health and well-being.

- **Get positive influences that challenge you to level up**

Surround yourself with supportive and positive people who encourage and uplift you. Seek mentors who can provide guidance, advice, and inspiration. You are not alone on this journey. You need like-minded friends and supporters.

Try new activities and experiences that challenge you. Each success will boost your confidence. Take calculated risks to build resilience and confidence in handling uncertainty. View mistakes as opportunities to learn and grow rather than as failures. Look back on them to find where you went wrong and work on your weaknesses.

- **Be empathic**

Practice empathy and understanding toward others, as this can improve your social interactions. You know how you need to recognize your faults and limitations; you need to recognize other people's limitations as well. Practice being assertive in expressing your needs and opinions while respecting others. Improve your communication skills by actively listening to others and engaging in meaningful conversations.

- **Regularly acknowledge and celebrate your achievements**

No matter how small your success may seem, acknowledge it and reward yourself for reaching milestones and accomplishing certain goals. The rewards don't have to be expensive, but something that makes you happy.

Don't hesitate to talk to your parents so you can seek help from a therapist or counselor if you're struggling with confidence or self-esteem issues. You can also utilize community resources such as workshops, seminars, and support groups.

By incorporating these practices into your daily life, you can build a strong foundation of confidence that will help you navigate the challenges of puberty and achieve your goals.

Conclusion

Well done, girl!

You made it to the end of this book, and I must commend you for doing such a fantastic job. You've taken this significant step toward understanding the changes happening to your body, emotions, and life in general. You should be proud of yourself for being curious and courageous at such a young age.

Before I leave you to start implementing all you've learned so far, I have a few words for you.

As you move forward, remember to embrace all the changes happening to your body and mind. Don't be hard on yourself; these changes are natural and what makes you unique. Also, take care of your body by practicing good hygiene, eating balanced meals, exercising regularly, and getting enough sleep.

I understand that your emotions might feel messed up and overwhelming sometimes. Instead of letting your emotions control you, you can find healthy ways to express and manage them. Examples include talking to someone, journaling, and engaging in activities you love. Remember, it's okay to experience a range of emotions during this phase; it's all part of growing up.

Ensure you talk to people you trust, such as your parents, friends, or any trusted adult. By sharing your thoughts and feelings, you'll feel understood and supported, making the weight feel lighter and easier to carry.

Embrace your strengths and celebrate your successes. Each challenge you overcome and every step you take to understand yourself better builds your confidence.

Stay curious and keep learning about your wonderful body. Check in with your support group often and be open to new discussions. If you have questions, reach out to your mom or any trusted adult who has experienced puberty. The more you know about puberty, the better you'll be at navigating the phase. Be patient and kind to yourself, as everyone's experience is different, and that's perfectly okay.

If you found this book helpful, share it with your friends. You can also leave a review to share your experience with other tweens looking for support and guidance through their own journey. By sharing your experiences, you're helping others feel less alone and more empowered.

Everybody needs a friend. This book is the friend that will support you through the stages of puberty. I'm glad that you've found this friend, and I promise it's a nice one.

Remember, puberty is just one part of your incredible journey. You have the strength, knowledge, and support to navigate it and get on with the next stage.

Keep believing in yourself and remember that you are never alone—you've got this book! Thank you for taking this journey with me. I'm so proud of you and excited about all the amazing things you'll accomplish.

Stay blessed!

A Respectful Request

I hope you enjoyed reading! Please share your story by leaving an **Amazon review**.

Reviews are the lifeblood of any author's career, and for a humbly independent writer like me, every review helps tremendously.

Even if it's only a sentence or two (although the longer the better!), it will be very helpful.

Please scan the below QR code to leave your review now.

Alternatively, you can visit:
www.bit.ly/review-puberty

Thank you.

A FREE GIFT TO OUR READERS

For being our valued reader, we are offering you 4 books absolutely FREE today.

What You'll Get:

1. **11 Essential Life Skills** Every Child Needs to Learn Before Leaving Home

2. How to **Be A Calm Parent** Even When Your Child Drives You Crazy

3. 15 Tips to **Build Self-Esteem and Confidence** in Teen Boys & Girls

4. **Anxiety Help** for Teenagers

Please scan the below QR code to download now.

Alternatively, you can visit:
www.thementorbucket.com/gift-puberty

MORE RECOMMENDED BOOKS

LIFE SKILLS FOR TWEENS WORKBOOK

How to Cook, Clean, Solve Problems, and Develop Self-Esteem, Confidence, and More

(Essential Life Skills Every Pre-Teen Needs but Doesn't Learn in School)

Get more details here:
www.thementorbucket.com/life-skills-tweens

ANGER MANAGEMENT WORKBOOK FOR KIDS

50+ Fun and Engaging Activities to Help Children Regain Control and Become Calmer and Happier

Get more details here:
www.thementorbucket.com/anger-kids

WANT TO READ MORE?

Before I close, I recommend you to read our other books in the series. These books are written especially for tweens, teens, and their parents. You'll find them very helpful.

**Get more details here:
www.thementorbucket.com/resources**

www.ingramcontent.com/pod-product-compliance
Lightning Source LLC
Chambersburg PA
CBHW071201120626
46546CB00006B/2368